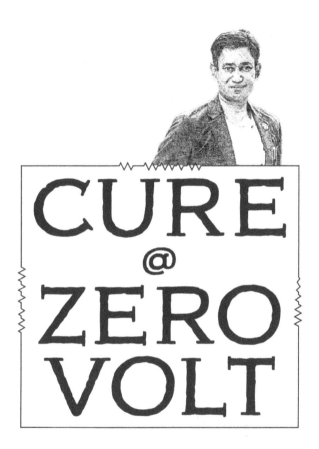

CURE @ ZERO VOLT

Dr. Biswaroop Roy Chowdhury

◉ DIAMOND BOOKS

India Office:
C/o India Book of Records
B-121, 2nd Floor, Greenfields,
Faridabad -120003 (Haryana),
India
Ph.: +91-9312286540

Malaysia Office:
C/o Bishwaroop International Healing
& Research
PT 573, Lot 15077 Jalan Tuanku
Munawir,
70000 Negeri Sembilan, Malaysia
Tel: +6012-2116089

Vietnam Office:
C/o Vietnam Book of Records
148 Hong Ha Street
9 Award, Phu Nhuan District,
Ho Chi Minh City, Vietnam
- Hotline: (+84) 903710505

Switzerland Office:
C/o Nigel Kingsley
Kraftwerkstr. 95, ch-5465, Mellikon,
Switzerland
Tel: 0041 79 222 2323

FOLLOW ME

Facebook: https://www.facebook.com/drbrc.official/
Twitter: https://twitter.com/drbrcofficial
Bitchute: https://www.bitchute.com/channel/drbiswarooproychowdhury/
Instagram: https://www.instagram.com/dr.biswarooproychowdhury/
Telegram: https://t.me/drbiswarooproychowdhury
Email: biswaroop@biswaroop.com
Website: www.biswaroop.com
Video Channel: www.coronakaal.tv

Research : Rachna Sharma
Graphics Designer: Shankar Singh Koranga, Swapan Banik
Video Translation: Narvijay Yadav

Published by
Diamond Pocket Books
X-30, Okhla Industrial Area, New Delhi-110020
Ph: 011-40712100   email: sales@dpb.in   website: www.diamondbook.in

Dedication

Dedicated to my angel daughter Ivy,

loving wife Neerja

&

caring parents

Shri Bikash Roy Chowdhury

Shrimati Lila Roy Chowdhury

CONTENTS

SECTION - I

SECTION - II

SECTION -I

CHAPTER -1

Cure through Medical Engineering

If you are aware of the 2017 noble prize for medicine, you will quickly understand that disturbing the circadian rhythm of the body leads to the manifestation of all possible lifestyle diseases. Even for infectious diseases, disturbance in the circadian rhythm creates a ground by lowering the immunity of the body. Circadian rhythm is essentially our body clock. Our body is designed to run in an optimum manner and in the most efficient fashion only if various hormonal changes follow a certain routine in a 24-hour cycle. For instance, the production of melatonin is expected to increase after sunset, whereas your body temperature should drop to its lowest towards the middle of the night. Some other changes that occur in the body to maintain the best health are indicated in the diagram below.

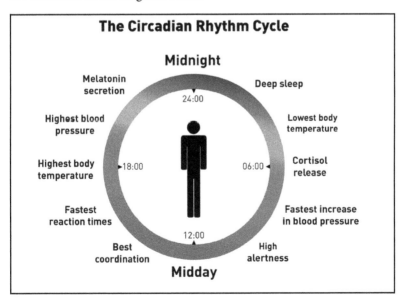

Any deviation from the set rules of the body clock leads to all kinds of illnesses. This means that the degree of your illness is directly proportional to the amount of deviation in your circadian rhythm.

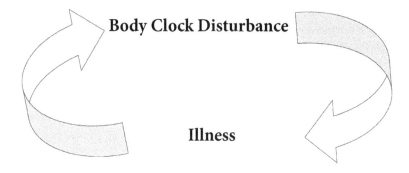

Body Clock Disturbance

Illness

Does that also mean that by correcting your circadian rhythm, you could possibly cure all kinds of diseases? My answer is a delightful Yes! We have seen remarkable results of cures through correcting the circadian rhythm in all kinds of diseases including diabetes, hypertension, heart diseases, arthritis, cancer, kidney failure. Ground breaking results are seen even in juvenile diseases like thalassemia, for which in modern medical literature, not even a single case of reversal of illness is recorded till now. However, we have with us more than 100 thalassemic children who were once dependent on blood transfusion. In such case of Umaija Haseen, a year and nine-month-old baby from Dhaka (Bangladesh), who was diagnosed to be thalassemia positive at the age of 5 months and was dependent on blood transfusion since then. After making certain changes in her daily routine, in

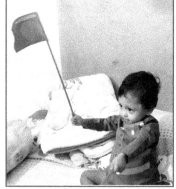

accordance with our understanding of correcting the circadian clock, the haemoglobin jumped from 4.8g/dl to 10.2g/dl within a span of just one month. And all the typical symptoms of thalassemia like continuous crying and irritating behaviour vanished. This happened without any blood transfusion.

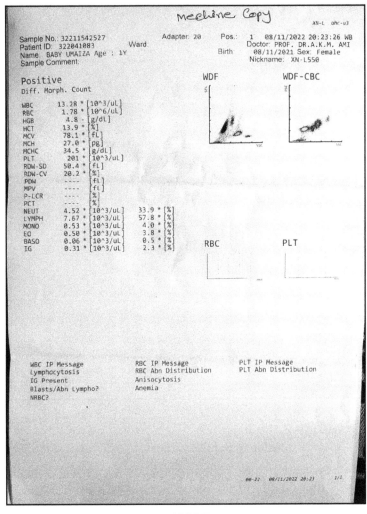

BEFORE

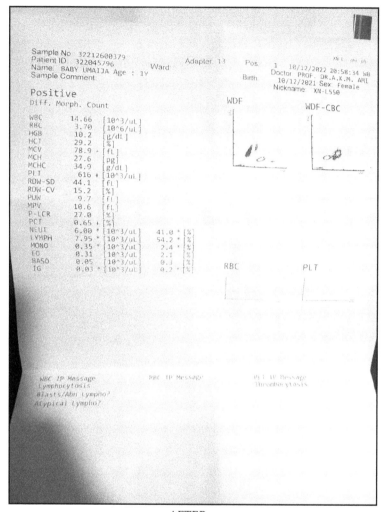

Sample No 32212600379
Patient ID 322045796
Name BABY UMAIJA Age : 1Y   Ward   Adapter. 13   Pos.
Sample Comment:

Positive
Diff. Morph. Count

WBC	14.66	[10^3/uL]			
RBC	3.70	[10^6/uL]			
HGB	10.2	[g/dL]			
HCT	29.2	[%]			
MCV	78.9	[fL]			
MCH	27.6	[pg]			
MCHC	34.9	[g/dL]			
PLT	616	[10^3/uL]			
RDW-SD	44.1	[fL]			
RDW-CV	15.2	[%]			
PDW	9.7	[fL]			
MPV	10.6	[fL]			
P-LCR	27.0	[%]			
PCT	0.65	[%]			
NEUT	6.00	[10^3/uL]	41.0	[%]	
LYMPH	7.95	[10^3/uL]	54.2	[%]	
MONO	0.35	[10^3/uL]	2.4	[%]	
EO	0.31	[10^3/uL]	2.1	[%]	
BASO	0.05	[10^3/uL]	0.3	[%]	
IG	0.03	[10^3/uL]	0.2	[%]	

WBC IP Message
Lymphocytosis
Blasts/Abn Lympho?
Atypical Lympho?

RBC IP Message

PLT IP Message
Thrombocytosis

AFTER

The results are so baffling that the medical council and various health authorities decided to give a blind eye to it, conveniently assuming the results are all doctored.

To read more similar success stories, read my book "Cure for Blood Disorders".

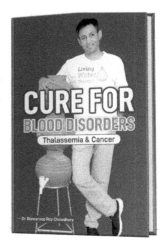

We have seen significant positive results among a wide spectrum of diseases within 72 hours of adopting our recommendation-based model of Circadian Triangle (Check the result of one of our recently concluded Cure @ 72 hours program ahead in this book).

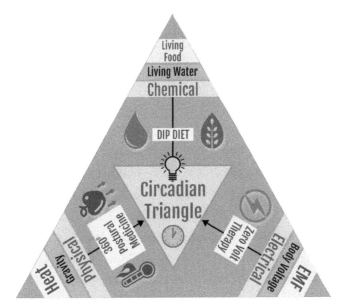

To understand my model of the 'Circadian Triangle', consider the three medical conditions.

1. Heart attack

2. Cardiac arrest

3. Coma

All the above often lead to death. Cardiac arrest is essentially the result of electrical failure of the body. However, on the other hand, a heart attack is something to do with a plaque (blockage) that can be seen as a physical clot formation, whereas a coma, let's say due to very low blood sugar; can be called a chemical imbalance of the body.

Our body functions in 3 different planes.

1. The physical body, like the structure and the location of various organs, is influenced directly by the force of gravity and the temperature of the environment.

2. The Chemical body, like the hormonal balance, the composition of minerals and vitamins and the chemistry of the blood greatly depend on the kind, quantity, and timing of what you eat and drink.

3. The electrical body has everything to do with your connectivity and conductivity with the earth.

To balance the chemical body, I have been recommending, my mathematical model-based "DIP diet" since 2014. It has almost an immediate impact on primary medical conditions including diabetes, hypertension, obesity, etc. To know about it, you can go through the Case Study – (Reversal of Type 1 Diabetes Using Plant-Based Diet *Journal of the Science of Healing Outcomes, Jan 2021 (Vol 13, No. 50)*, Clinical trial of the DIP Diet by All India Institute of Ayurveda (Under Ministry of AYUSH, Govt. of India) *Ctri/2018/12/016654*, read several of my books including "Last days of Diabetes" and

"The Diabetes-free World" or search for thousands of videos on DIP diet, uploaded on the internet, by my successful patients.

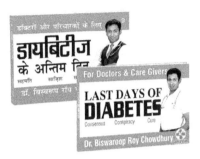 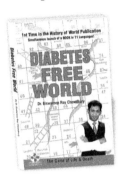

To balance the physical body, I have developed a law of gravity and a heat-based "GRAD System". The observational study done on the GRAD system proved its effectiveness in reversing kidney failure and freeing the patient from dialysis dependency. The GRAD system has been the foundation protocol at our HIIMS chain of hospitals and is now adopted by other hospitals in India, Nepal, Vietnam and Malaysia.

To learn about it, read my books "360⁰ Postural Medicine" & "The End of Transplant".

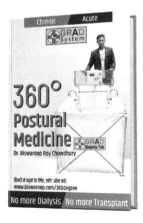 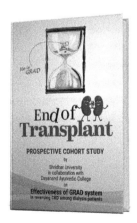

I paid attention to balancing the electrical aspect of the body only in the last several months while solving the puzzle of thalassemia. I discovered, that within a few minutes of putting our body at Zero Voltage, the disappearance of chronic inflammation and a measurable improvement in terms of pain and symptomatic relief is seen in the patient.

Conclusively, my protocol for solving the problem of human health crisis has nothing to do with drugs or surgery. It's all about the law of gravity, heat, the flow of electrons, and the mathematical model of nutrition. Essentially using the principles of engineering to resolve health issues, is called Medical Engineering - a field that got into prominence only in the last decade.

My innovations like the DIP diet and the GRAD system are elaborately explained in many of my books and literally through thousands of videos on social media.

Through this book, I present my latest innovation i.e. "The Zero Volt therapy" especially to correct the electrical balance of the body. Failing to do so, often leads to various chronic inflammatory conditions including heart diseases and cancer.

CHAPTER -2

Electro Magnetic Field - The Invisible Enemy

(This chapter is taken from the lecture of "Zero Volt Therapy" certification course).

Let me share with you a couple of flashbacks before we begin.

During the Lockdown period in 2020, when an atmosphere of fear and death prevailed, and in this period common colds, coughs and fevers were termed COVID, and patients suffering from these were placed in quarantine. People were so scared that they preferred to jump off to death from the hospitals and their own house terraces than, face the hardships after being termed as COVID Positive. During this time our N.I.C.E (Network of Influenza Cure Experts) and W.I.S.E. experts who had taken their 3-months online training in medical nutrition from Lincoln University Malaysia and Shridhar University, together as health practitioners and paramedics, tried to implement what they had learned in medical nutrition training like **DIP Diet** and the **3-Step Flu Diet**. These two types of diet were a mathematical model of nutrition, a formula for taking nutrients that worked wonders whether it was the 3-step Flu diet of taking coconut water and citrus fruit juice or the DIP Diet of Plate 1 formula.

Millions of people who followed the DIP Diet & 3-Step Flu Diet became better and then, they realized that it was not COVID but actually Flu. Because of the fear in the minds of people, a common medical condition was perceived as a dangerous disease. At this crucial time, together N.I.C.E & W.I.S.E experts helped millions of people to come out of that fear.

> **NIN, Ministry of Ayush did an observational study on 3 Step Flu diet and recommended it in the prevention and cure of mild & sever cases of COVID-19**
>
> *To read the observation study, go to*
> *www.biswaroop.com/ayush*

Still, this nutrition therapy could not reach many others who in the midst of such a fearful atmosphere had already reached the hospitals and were given remidesivir, lopinavir, ritonavir, plasma therapy, hydroxychloroquine, etc. These were banned medicines (and banned till date). At that time such drugs were given to people and their side effects hit so badly that most patients actually died and those who managed to survive suffered from kidney failure, liver failure, heart disease, or they were troubled with diabetes. It was not a treatment; it was just a way or a method to cause or create disease among people. It was a conspiracy, a PLANDEMIC.

Last year i.e. in 2021, I observed that kidney failure patients were exponentially increasing and upon digging into their history, we found out that they were the same who in the name of COVID had received medical treatment. In such cases, the only alternative they had was that they should go for a kidney transplant or go for dialysis. Some of them had already started the process of dialysis.

During this period, the 'Emergency and Pain Management Training' by Sridhar University Rajasthan was introduced. The training had an aim that the exponential growth of the disease that has set in because of the side-effects of those banned medications – such patients should get relief. Those who joined this training and became certified EPM

Paramedics supported and extended their help in the recovery of these patients.

Hospital & Institute of Integrated Medical Sciences (HIIMS) and its branches were also opened where such patients could reach to get treatment. The idea was that we need to provide an overall education, where people learn while sitting at home and get cured. The results were good.

With the help of Hot Water Immersion, the 360 Degrees Postural Medicines and the Head-Down Tilt, people are recovering and getting cured.

So the crux of the matter is that our health has three dimensions. And, these three dimensions together converge into what is called the **Circadian Triangle**.

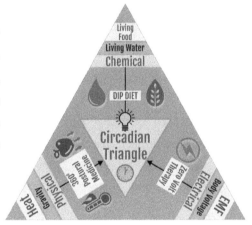

The First dimension of the Circadian Triangle is the **'Chemical Aspect'** of the body. You are made of chemicals and the balance and imbalance of the chemicals in the body depends on the fact whether you are ill or not. If you are ill and your chemical balance is disrupted, you can use the 3-Step Flu Diet or the DIP Diet to help you revive and regain your chemical balance. This has been implemented successfully by our N.I.C.E., W.I.S.E., and EPM Paramedics. They witnessed how the chemical balance through the DIP Diet and 3-Step Flu helped in getting rid of pain and discomfort with rapid speed. This is one angle; just one aspect of your health.

The second dimension of the Circadian Triangle is the **'Physical Aspect'**. This has been widely used since last year and involves your body's structure, your bone design, your body skin, and the outer covering of the body. Any disruption or imbalance in the physical aspect of the body can be rectified with the help of the GRAD system. The GRAD system includes Hot Water Immersion, Lower Leg Hot Water Immersion, Head down Tilt, etc. Using this technique we witnessed how irrecoverable patients had recovered.

If you recall, the real pandemic that happened last year, was actually the side effects of the medicines that led to the exponential increase in illnesses and chronic diseases.

Now, in 2022, we are struggling with a strange situation in which even you must have noticed that people while walking or dancing or even while exercising in the gym are suddenly dying. They are dying while driving a bus, or while getting married.

Apparently, they are dying without any reason; even 13-year-olds are dying suddenly. This phenomenon is noticed not only in India but throughout the world. Especially, this phenomenon is seen with only those people who got vaccinated for COVID-19. And this is not an unusual thing, this is something we already knew. Let's recall, all those who know me before or since 2020; in the month of August through various web conferences and physical conferences we kept spreading awareness about vaccines and that the vaccines are being manufactured with the sole purpose of depopulation. Corresponding

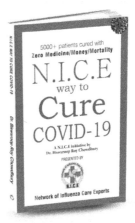

to it, we also launched the Book, 'N.I.C.E way to cure COVID-19' in the month of October 2020.

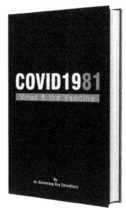

After that in the month of November, on the occasion of Rajiv Dixit Jayanti, we launched another book 'COVID 1981, Virus & the Vaccine'.

In this book, we clearly mentioned, that the COVID Vaccine, which most of the population has already received, will lead to an increased number of sudden deaths and will also see an increased number of cases of infertility, diabetes, and many other kinds of maladies.

Today, we are actually standing in that same position where we are witnessing all these fall-outs of the side effects widely.

If anyone has even the slightest doubt regarding whatever is happening around them, such as people dying, diseases increasing exponentially, infertility increasing, impotency increasing, and feeling there is no role of the vaccine then take a look at the below-given slides.

Comparative risk of thrombosis with thrombocytopenia syndrome or thromboembolic events associated with different covid-19 vaccines: international network cohort study from five European countries and the US
Li X, Burn E, Duarte-Salles T, Yin C, Reich C, Delmestri A et al.BMJ 2022; 379 :e071594 doi:10.1136/bmj-2022-071594

Relationship between blood clots and COVID-19 vaccines: A literature review.
Atyabi SMH, Rommasi F, Ramezani MH, Ghane Ezabadi MF, Arani MA, Sadeghi MH, Ahmed MM, Rajabi A, Dehghan N, Sohrabi A, Seifi M, Nasiri MJ.Open Life Sci. 2022 Apr 26;17(1):401-415. doi: 10.1515/biol-2022-0035

These are all the research papers that are clear-cut evidence and prove that those who have taken the vaccine get blood clots, and these clots result in heart attack, cardiac arrest, and hemorrhages. These research papers can be downloaded from this link: www.biswaroop.com/zvtbook for a deep study of the research. Apart from this, the biggest study in the world on the COVID Vaccine was conducted in Israel, where more than 4 million people who had received vaccination participated in the study. Those who received vaccines had 51% increased chances of a cardiac syndrome than those non-vaccinated. This research paper was released in the world's most prestigious journal called 'Nature', in April 2022.

Increased emergency cardiovascular events among under-40 population in Israel during vaccine rollout and third COVID-19 wave.
Sun, C.L.F., Jaffe, E. & Levi, R.Sci Rep 12, 6978 (2022). https://doi.org/10.1038/s41598-022-10928-z

Another research paper was released in the month of September 2022 by Dr. Aseem Malhotra, an Indian-origin British cardiologist who used to speak in favor of vaccines. After his father's death, he got a post-mortem done and in the autopsy report, he found out that the cause of his death was nothing but the vaccine's side effect. After this, he further deepened his research, which was published in a prestigious journal, called the 'Journal of Insulin Resistance'.

Curing the pandemic of misinformation on COVID-19 mRNA vaccines through real evidence-based medicine - Part 1Aseem Malhotra
*Journal of Insulin Resistance	Vol 5, No 1	a71 |*

Recently in the month of November 2022, a 'German Study' was released, which was done on all those dying suddenly while at work or the gym or doing any other daily routine chore.

German Study: Autopsy-based histopathological characterization of myocarditis after anti-SARS-CoV-2-vaccination
Clin Res Cardiol (2022). Schwab, C., Domke, L.M., Hart-mann, L. et al.https://doi.o rg/10.1007/s00392-022-02129-5

> **Thailand Study: Cardiovascular Manifestation of the BNT162b2 mRNA COVID-19 Vaccine in Adolescents.**
>
> *Mansanguan, S.; Charunwatthana, P.; Piyaphanee, W.; Dechkhajorn, W.; Poolcharoen, A.; Mansanguan, C. Trop. Med. Infect. Dis. 2022, 7, 196. https://doi.org/10.3390/tropicalmed7080196*

There are many similar studies that have been conducted but the ones quoted here are really large-scale and authentic studies, which prove with absolute clarity that all those who got vaccinated are in a very dangerous situation i.e. sudden death without any warning.

In this chapter, we will focus on identifying the problem. We faced a certain problem in 2020 which was fear or fear-mongering. In 2021, the widespread illness was the side-effect of the treatment protocols in the name of Covid. Its side effects were kidney failure, and liver failure in dangerous proportions – as noticed in 2021.

And now, the situation is, people are dying of sudden deaths! Behind this situation is one of the enemies I have been telling you about since 2020 when the vaccine was not even brought in. The vaccine is one enemy and another enemy seemingly harmless and invisible is EMF i.e. Electromagnetic Field, specially ever since 5G is released.

At this point, comes into picture the third dimension - the **'Electrical Aspect'**. Your body has some electrical properties or we can say your body is like an electrical gadget. Have you noticed that a doctor checks you with a stethoscope through which he listens to your heartbeat? Since your body is emanating electrical signals, with the help of various diagnostic tools doctors try to read or understand your electro-cardio signals as ECG or your brain's electrical signals i.e. EEG. Based on your body's electrical signals the diagnosis is done.

Currently, we are fighting with two major issues i.e. side effects of the Covid-19 vaccine and the second one is 5G, which is an invisible enemy but can still be seen in the form of day-to-day activities, which are increasingly becoming digitalized. Even money or currency is getting digital. Children's education is getting online for the past three years when they were made to stay glued to the mobiles, surrounded by electromagnetic fields for 8 to 10 hours. We need to understand that the electromagnetic field is invisible. Anything that is invisible is perceived to be not dangerous, for example, the gravitational force is invisible and it is not dangerous. Air is invisible, but that also works on our body and is not dangerous.

One thing that has been ignored so far is that the human body has an electrical field. Let us understand this fact with the help of two magnets. During childhood, you must have done this activity. Place two magnets closer with the same poles facing each other. You would see that they repel each other. This happens due to an invisible field between the two magnets which results in repelling i.e. one is interfering with the magnetic field of the other. This is an example of a magnetic field that you already know. What I am doing is simply reminding you about the existence of a magnetic field.

In the same way, our earth has a geomagnetic field that can be demonstrated through a compass. The needle of the compass changes direction with your motion and always points the north. Another example of geo-compass is found in animals and birds when they migrate from one place to another with a precise understanding of direction. Unlike us, they do not have a google map. They just follow the geomagnetic field of the earth. So the earth is an entity that has a magnetic field and you also have a magnetic field. Even man-made tools, electrical equipment, mobiles, television, camera, and Wi-Fi - all have their own electromagnetic field. Even plants have their own electromagnetic field. Just like magnets, when they come closer they affect each other and can be noticed physically when they attract or repel each other. In the same way, the moment I bring a plant near me, its electromagnetic field overlaps with my electromagnetic field.

Similarly, our cell phones or mobiles when switched on radiate their own electromagnetic fields which overlap with each other. Take another example of you sitting in a room. Look around yourself. There are various electromagnetic fields in the room. There is TV, Wi-Fi, tube lights, and cell phone, each having an electromagnetic field that gets interfered with and overlaps. When they overlap they somehow affect each other, in a positive or negative manner. This means when you are in a jungle, surrounded by trees, their electromagnetic fields overlap with yours. However, an interesting fact is that when two natural electromagnetic fields overlap or interfere with each other, they do no harm. But the electromagnetic fields of man-made products impact us negatively.

Let me explain with another example. When you talk on your mobile for 20 minutes or more, the temperature of your ear increases by one degree. After every 20 minutes, the temperature keeps on increasing. You can feel your ear getting warmer. This means you have created an artificial fever. When you have this fever for a longer duration, you develop a condition called tinnitus. In this state, people hear a ringing sound in the ear. This is called the micro-wave hearing, a hearing range available to the sufferer, which otherwise is not audible to the human race, normally.

If you continue to create such a fever, then your ears will start catching other kinds of signals also. The echo you will feel becomes very distracting and you feel disturbed and not able to concentrate or sleep. There will be constant irritation. You must have noticed that over a period of time especially with prolonged exposure to mobile radiation, you feel lethargy, laziness, weakness, and fatigue. This is because you are unknowingly surrounded by radiation. Even though your body keeps functioning but it is causing clear-cut damage. Let us understand which radiations are harmful and which ones are harmless. In order to go deep into research, you can study this paper and understand it.

The paper is available at www.biswaroop.com/zvtbook

"Adverse Influence of Radio Frequency Background on Trembling Aspen Seedlings: Preliminary Observations"

Katie Haggerty, International Journal of Forestry Research, vol. 2010, Article ID 836278, 7 pages, 2010.

Many of us have the habit of keeping our mobile phone in the shirt pocket closer to the heart, or in the front pockets of our trousers. In case they keep it in their pant pocket, it may cause infertility. Research proves that 'men with erectile dysfunction are more likely to have mobile phones in the front pocket of their pants'.

> **Men with erectile dysfunction are 2.6 times more likely to have mobile phones in the front pocket of their pants.**
>
> *Abstracts of the World Meeting on Sexual Medicine. Chicago, Illinois, USA. August 26-30, 2012. A. Moore, K. Flynn, J. Lai Published 2012. Medicine. The journal of sexual medicine.*

Similarly, those who complained of heart palpitations were found to be keeping their mobile phones in their shirt pocket.

This means that you need to remember not to keep the mobile near your skin. You can take a bag to keep your mobile or else you can keep it in flight mode and switch off the bluetooth and then keep the mobile in either your shirt or pant pocket. Remember, just because electromagnetic waves are invisible, does not mean that they are not working on you and are not dangerous!

We can now glance through the electromagnetic spectrum.

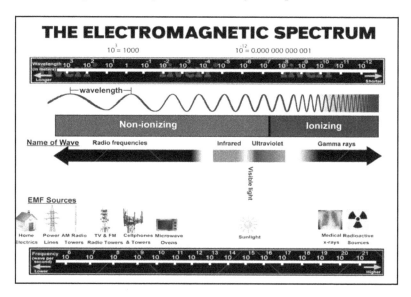

You may notice that electromagnetic waves will enter your house through various sources and at different wavelengths like power lines, electrical equipment, and home appliances like ovens – all these produce electromagnetic waves. Just like the waves produced by the sun that reaches your house, medical equipment that produces waves (X-Ray machines), and radioactive forces that produce electromagnetic waves. Out of all these what is natural is the sunlight and apart from sunlight, the rest is only harming your body.

In case you are wondering if the mobile phone is so dangerous that it creates infertility and impotency and brings many changes to the body, then how come you didn't know all this before or no one told you? Dear all, you were told! But you took it very lightly.

Whenever you purchase a new mobile phone, there is a leaflet or a user manual that comes with it. How many of you read it or tried reading it? And in case you read it, for example, if you read the Samsung mobile's manual it is mentioned that whenever you receive a call you should keep the phone 1.5 cm away from your ear because it can be carcinogenic. And if you can't find your leaflet then I have collected all sorts of leaflets which can be downloaded through this link from my website: www.biswaroop.com/cellphonefever.

Once you will read the leaflets, you will understand that whatever I am telling you here through this book is already known to the world. But they have told you in such a light and mild way that you never paid attention. However, if you do not pay attention that does not mean that it's not harming you. It is continuously harming you. So out of your convenience, you ignored the warning, but this ignorance or neglect will cost you heavily.

You are all well aware that you are surrounded by bacteria and viruses all the time, but most of them are friendly viruses and bacteria, and only a few of them are harmful. Similarly, everywhere you go, you are surrounded by an electromagnetic field. Some of these electromagnetic fields are nature-made for example geomagnetic fields, also known as gravity, EMF from plants, sunlight, moonlight, etc. What nature has made for you harmonizes with your body and is good for you. However, what man has made is not good for you because these EMFs are most of the time or all the time 'Polarized'.

Polarized EMF goes inside your body and causes oscillation of free radicals. The basic purpose of free radicals in your body is that they help in building immunity, which keeps a check on the diseases in your body. What happens with the oscillation of free radicals is that it disrupts the cell's electrochemical balance and when this happens, it invites diseases like cancer. So you need to understand that mobiles and other man-made equipment like microwave ovens, or X-Rays that give out electromagnetic fields are very damaging in nature because of polarization.

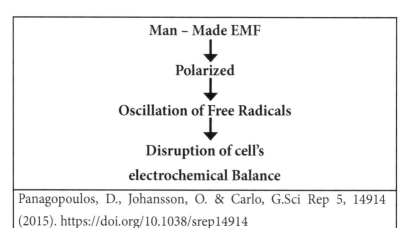

Man – Made EMF

↓

Polarized

↓

Oscillation of Free Radicals

↓

Disruption of cell's electrochemical Balance

Panagopoulos, D., Johansson, O. & Carlo, G.Sci Rep 5, 14914 (2015). https://doi.org/10.1038/srep14914

Further in-depth knowledge can be accessed through the research paper quoted as a reference in the previous picture.

I summarized some points for your easy reference on the harmful effects of the man-made electromagnetic fields from mobile phones, X-rays, microwaves, etc, and are shown below:

Cell phone radiation causes
- **Reduced sperm count**
- **Reduced sperm motility**
- **Reduced sperm morphology**
- **Reduced level of testosterone**

The research papers based on which I summarized the above points are shown below:

---

1. **Effect of cell phone usage on semen analysis in men attending infertility clinic: an observational study. Agarwal A, Deepinder F, Sharma RK, Ranga G, Li J. Fertil Steril. 2008 Jan;89(1):124-8. doi: 10.1016/j. fertnstert.2007.01.166. Epub 2007 May 4. PMID: 17482179.**
2. **The effects of radiofrequency electromagnetic radiation on sperm function. Houston BJ, Nixon B, King BV, De Iuliis GN, Aitken RJ. Reproduction. 2016 Dec;152(6):R263-R276. doi: 10.1530/REP-16-0126. Epub 2016 Sep 6. PMID: 27601711.**
3. **The effect of pulsed 900-MHz GSM mobile phone radiation on the acrosome reaction, head morphometry and zona binding of human spermatozoa. Falzone N, Huyser C, Becker P, Leszczynski D, Franken DR Int J Androl. 2011 Feb;34(1):20-6. doi: 10.1111/j.1365-2605.2010.01054.x. PMID: 20236367.**

> **4. Effects of mobile phone radiation on serum testosterone in Wistar albino rats. Meo SA, Al-Drees AM, Husain S, Khan MM, Imran MB. Saudi Med J. 2010 Aug;31(8):869-73. PMID: 20714683.**

While we are talking about male fertility and how it is negatively impacted by mobile phones, this is not just limited to the use of mobiles. Wi-Fi also plays a major role in causing male infertility.

> ## Wi-fi can reduce male fertility
> Use of laptop computers connected to the internet through Wi-Fi decreases human sperm motility and increases sperm DNA fragmentation, Conrado Avendaño, Ariela Mata, César A. Sanchez Sarmiento, Gustavo F. Doncel, Fertility and Sterility. Volume 97, Issue 1,2012,Pages 39-45.e2,ISSN 0015-0282.

While in this chapter we are discussing the problems created by Wi-Fi or the harmful effect of EMF, the solution is discussed in the next chapter.

You must have noticed that you are surrounded by invisible electrical charges all the time. This is quite noticeable sometimes when you happen to touch a door knob and you suddenly get a mild shock making you pull back your hand abruptly. This means that your body along with other objects is surrounded by an electrical charge.

This can be easily seen through an experiment by rubbing a wooden pencil against your shirt. Now bring this charged pencil near some pieces of shredded paper. They will stick to the pencil. Another DIY (do it yourself) example is to rub an inflated balloon against a cloth and then bring this charged balloon near your hair. Hair strands get attracted and stick to the balloon.

These simple examples prove that we are surrounded by electrical charges all the time. Even though invisible to us they have an impact on our bodies. Similarly, prolonged use of mobiles and Wi-Fi disrupts brain functioning, causing depression. The brain generally releases various hormones like Serotonin, Dopamine, Endorphins, Oxytocin, Melatonin, etc, which regulate calmness, happiness, and good sleep in the body. EMF from mobile disrupts the regulation of the above-mentioned hormones and creates stress in the body resulting in the production of Cortisol hormone which leads to depression and anxiety.

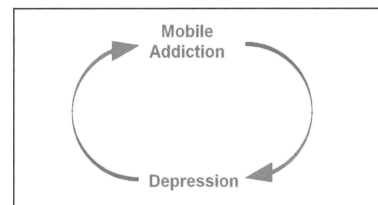

Mobile Addiction

Depression

Microwave frequency electromagnetic fields (EMFs) produce widespread neuropsychiatric effects including depression. Pall ML. J Chem Neuroanat. 2016 Sep;75(Pt B):43-51. doi: 10.1016/j.jchemneu.2015.08.001. Epub 2015 Aug 21. PMID: 26300312.

When you are depressed your mobile addiction increases, which in turn again increases depression. This forms a vicious cycle, thus aggravating the problem without us realizing it.

All these problems are not just limited only to mobile phones. Cell phone towers are also a source of EMFs and various research studies found that those who reside near cell phone towers are more prone to anxiety, depression, fatigue, tiredness, and lethargy.

Cellphone Tower Distance **Depression fatigue**

Investigation on the health of people living near mobile telephone relay stations: I/Incidence according to distance and sex. Santini R, Santini P, Danze JM, Le Ruz P, Seigne M. Pathol Biol (Paris). 2002 Jul; 50(6):369-73. French. doi: 10.1016/s0369-8114(02)00311-5. Erratum in: Pathol Biol (Paris). 2002 Dec; 50(10):621. PMID: 12168254.

Another concerning and alarming fact is that EMF exposure can increase the chances of miscarriage three times. That means pregnant women should restrict the use of mobile phones and if possible reduce their exposure to EMF or shield themselves from EMF. How can they shield themselves from EMF is discussed in the next chapter.

EMF exposure can increase the risk of miscarriage three times.

Exposure to Magnetic Field Non-Ionizing Radiation and the Risk of Miscarriage: A Prospective Cohort Study. Li, DK., Chen, H., Ferber, J.R. et al. Sci Rep 7, 17541 (2017). https://doi.org/10.1038/s41598-017-16623-8

EMF not only increases the chances of miscarriage among pregnant women but also impacts the growth and development of the child growing in the mother's womb. High EMF exposure damages the stem cells of the growing baby, which in turn hampers the growth of the brain cells leading to autism in children.

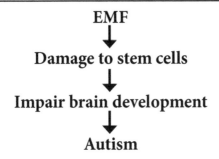

EMF

↓

Damage to stem cells

↓

Impair brain development

↓

Autism

Research on Correlation Between Autism, Cell Phones, and Wireless Computers by Tamara Mariea Martes 17 de abril de 2007. Genetic engineering and biotechnology news

In the last three years during PLANDEMIC, children were deliberately made to sit for online classes for more than 10 hours a day exposing them to high EMF. After the online classes since lockdown was imposed everywhere, children were engaged in online games prolonging their exposure to EMF. All this resulted in an increasing number of autism or auto-immune diseases among children.

I would also like to draw your attention to the fact that small children have delicate skin and bones so the EMF absorption is 60% higher than an average adult. A one-year-old baby absorbs 100% more EMF.

> ## 5-year-old absorbs 60% more radiation than an adult. One year old absorbs double the radiation
>
> Application of the Precautionary Approach to Mobile Phone Technology. Archived on 10 Sep 2010. The National Archives Govt of U.K.

This exposure disrupts the genetic composition in the children and damages their DNA structure. So the implication is not only making you sick but is a plan to turn the generations to be sick and handicapped.

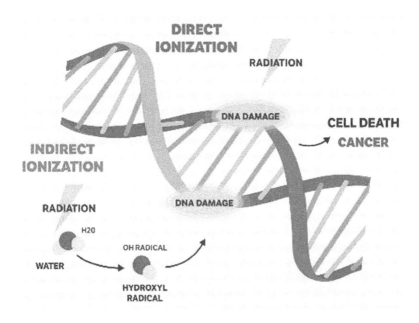

The plan to destroy our next generation starts from the womb of the mothers. EMF exposure in the womb leads to children being born Obese, Asthmatic, and suffering from attention deficit disorders.

EMF exposure in the womb
- **Obesity**
- **Asthma**
- **Attention problem**

1. A Prospective Study of In-utero Exposure to Magnetic Fields and the Risk of Childhood Obesity July 2012Scientific Reports 2(1):540 DOI:10.1038/srep00540 Source: PubMed

2. Maternal Exposure to Magnetic Fields During Pregnancy in Relation to the Risk of Asthma in Offspring. Li D, Chen H, Odouli R. Arch Pediatr Adolesc Med. 2011;165(10):945–950. doi: 10.1001/archpediatrics.2011.135

3. Maternal cell phone use during pregnancy and child behavioral problems in five birth cohorts. Birks L, Guxens M, Papadopoulou E, Alexander J, Ballester F, Estarlich M, Gallastegi M, Ha M, Haugen M, Huss A, Kheifets L, Lim H, Olsen J, Santa-Marina L, Sudan M, Vermeulen R, Vrijkotte T, Cardis E, Vrijheid M. Environ Int. 2017 Jul;104:122-131. doi: 10.1016/j.envint.2017.03.024. Epub 2017 Apr 7. PMID: 28392066; PMCID: PMC5506372.

Another study found that 10-year-old children absorb more radiation making them sick with various types of cancer. No wonder I am observing an increased number of parents approaching us for treatment of autoimmune diseases, autism, SMA, and cancer.

10-year-old child absorbs 153% more cellphone radiation than an adult

Exposure Limits: The underestimation of absorbed cell phone radiation, especially in children. Gandhi, Om & Morgan, L Lloyd & Salles, Alvaro & Han, Yueh-Ying & Herberman, Ronald & Davis, Devra. (2012) Electromagnetic biology and medicine. 31. 34-51. 10.3109/15368378.2011.622827.

Cellphone/wireless radiations are classified as class-B human carcinogens.

Exposure limits: the underestimation of absorbed cell phone radiation, especially in children. Gandhi OP, Morgan LL, de Salles AA, Han YY, Herberman RB, Davis DL , Electromagn Biol Med. 2012 Mar; 31(1):34-51. doi: 10.3109/15368378.2011.622827. Epub 2011 Oct 14. PMID: 21999884.

Just like cigarettes are classified as Class B human carcinogens and every single pack of cigarettes carries a 'cancer-causing' warning. A similar warning should be there on mobile phone packages too.

But since the mobile phone lobby is rich and powerful, all this information is kept under tight wraps. The information remained confined to research journals and could not reach the masses.

I however collated 7 such major studies to understand the gravity of the matter:

1. German study: This study found that those who are residing within 400 meters of cell phone towers were reported to be suffering more from cancer.

2. Israeli Study: This study also substantiated the fact that the closer the cell phone tower, the greater the chances of suffering from cancer.

3. Nearness to cell phone towers is also linked to childhood leukemia.

4. EMF causes DNA damage.

5. Cell phone radiation causes tumors on the same side of the head

6. Wi-Fi can cause cancer.

7. Interphone Study: The risk of a glioma increases by 40% with 1640 hours of mobile phone use.

German Study

Within 400 m of roof cell tower 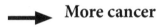 **More cancer**

The Influence of Being Physically Near to a Cell Phone Transmission Mast on the Incidence of Cancer. Horst Eger, Klaus Uwe Hagen, Birgitt Lucas, Peter Vogel, Helmut Voit Published in Umwelt·Medizin·Gesellschaft 17,4 2004,

---

Israeli study

Closer to cell tower ⟶ **More cancer**

Carcinogenicity of radiofrequency electromagnetic fields. Robert Baan Yann Grosse Béatrice Lauby-Secretan. Fatiha El Ghissassi Véronique Bouvard Lamia Benbrahim-Tallaa et al. The Lancet Oncology Volume 12, Issue 7, P624-626, July 01, 2011.

Cell tower is linked to childhood leukemia

Cancer incidence and mortality and proximity to TV towers. Hocking B, Gordon IR, Grain HL, Hatfield GE. Med J Aust. 1996 Dec 2-16;165(11-12):601-5. doi: 10.5694/j.1326-5377.1996.tb138661.x. Erratum in: Med J Aust 1997 Jan 20;166(2):80. PMID: 8985435.

EMF causes DNA damage

Impact of radiofrequency radiation on DNA damage and antioxidants in peripheral blood lymphocytes of humans residing in the vicinity of mobile phone base stations, Zothansiama, Mary Zosangzuali, Miriam Lalramdinpuii & Ganesh Chandra Jagetia (2017) Electromagnetic Biology and Medicine, 36:3, 295-305, DOI: 10.1080/15368378.2017.1350584

Cellphone radiation causes tumor on the same side of the head

Cell phones and brain tumors: a review including the long-term epidemiologic data. Khurana VG, Teo C, Kundi M, Hardell L, Carlberg M. Surg Neurol. 2009 Sep;72(3):205-14; discussion 214-5. doi: 10.1016/j.surneu.2009.01.019. Epub 2009 Mar 27. PMID: 19328536.

Wi-fi can cause cancer

Çiğ B, Nazıroğlu M. Investigation of the effects of distance from sources on apoptosis, oxidative stress and cytosolic calcium accumulation via TRPV1 channels induced by mobile phones and Wi-Fi in breast cancer cells. Biochim Biophys Acta. 2015 Oct;1848 (10 Pt B):2756-65. doi: 10.1016/j.bbamem.2015.02.013. Epub 2015 Feb 19. PMID: 25703814.

Interphone Study (IARC)

Risk of glioma increase by 40% with 1640 hrs of cell phone use

The above studies tell us about the physical manifestation of exposure to EMF. The following research papers highlight the damages on a mental level.

2.9 times higher risk of ADHD→mother with higher exposure to EMF

Adverse Fetal and Childhood Health Effect of In-Utero Exposure to Magnetic Fields Non-ionizing Radiation. Division of Research Kaiser Foundation Research Institute Kaiser Permanente, Oakland, California, Accessed August 15, 2019

You must have observed that cases of ADHD (Attention Deficit Hyperactivity Disorder) have increased in schools by almost three folds. The schools also have Wi-Fi and smart boards causing electromagnetic pollution and exposing children to harmful EMF. The school authorities like principals, teachers, etc can be made aware of this electrical pollution. You will be able to do so with more authority once you qualify as Zero Volt Therapy Experts (ZVTE), through the training initiated by the Research Institute of Complementary Health Sciences, Vietnam.

Moving on to the next study which revealed that EMF exposure is linked to childhood obesity. Another study highlighted how Wi-Fi can impair brain function.

EMF exposure is linked to childhood obesity

EMF Exposures in the Womb Can Lead to Childhood Obesity. Kaiser's De-Kun Li Second Prospective Study July 27, 2012, MicroWave News

---

Wi-Fi can impair brain function

Effects of 2.4 GHz radiofrequency radiation emitted from Wi-Fi equipment on microRNA expression in brain tissue. Dasdag S, Akdag MZ, Erdal ME, Erdal N, Ay OI, Ay ME, Yilmaz SG, Tasdelen B, Yegin K. Int J Radiat Biol. 2015 Jul;91(7):555-61. doi: 10.3109/09553002.2015.1028599. Epub 2015 May 20. PMID: 25775055.

All this while we focused on EMF radiations from mobile phones, iPad, and laptops. The laptop, as the name itself indicates, can be kept on a lap for easy working and accessibility. But this convenience costs us in the form of erectile dysfunction, infertility, impotency, etc.

Let's now discuss 'Blue Light'. Whether the blue light is from mobile, TV, laptop or iPad, it interferes with the Circadian Rhythm of our body, especially during the night. Circadian Rhythm refers to the biological clock. We all have a clock ingrained in our body that regulates different hormones according to the time of the day, for example, it induces sleep at night, and energizes and refreshes the body in the morning and during the day. This biological clock is termed Circadian Rhythm. The Circadian Rhythm gets disrupted more when exposed to blue light after sunset or at night. We all have developed a habit of surfing social media like Facebook, WhatsApp, Youtube, Instagram, etc, before going to sleep, exposing ourselves to blue light during a time when it should be avoided by all means. This interferes with the body's Circadian Rhythm and causes various diseases in the body. A more detailed study on blue light and its adverse effects will be taken up later, but for now, as a take-home message, you can avoid exposure to blue light by staying away from mobiles, computers, and TV screens at night.

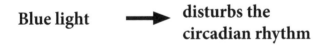

Another important example of EMF exposure is 'Ultrasound'. Would-be mothers are more exposed to EMF through ultrasound under the pretext of knowing the status of the growing fetus. Pregnancy in today's time is seen more as an illness rather than a natural process. Expecting mothers are made to visit hospitals, given various kinds of supplements and made to undergo numerous ultrasound scanning. All this is done to know the progress of the fetus and its healthy development. Even today in our country, more than 70% of the babies are delivered at home without any assistance from so-called modern health care system and they are all born healthy and strong.

Repeated ultrasound scans on pregnant women expose the fetus to dangerous EMF and owing to the vulnerability of the growing fetus to absorb a high level of radiation more harm is done at various genetic, mental, and physical levels. Such babies are born with various disabilities or develop various diseases like cancer in early childhood.

Therefore, pregnant women should minimize or avoid hospital visits and exposure to ultrasound as far as possible. Deliveries should be done at home rather than in the hospitals.

Let me elucidate how EMF exposure through ultrasound, CT Scans, mobile phones, or by any other means damages your body at the cellular level. Take a look at the picture:

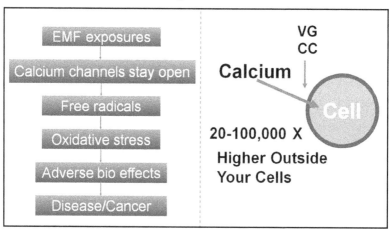

Human cells have Calcium ions in them and are also surrounded on the outside by a high concentration of Calcium ions. To maintain the equilibrium, Calcium ions enter and exit the cells through small openings or doors on the cell membrane known as 'Voltage-Gated Calcium-Channels'. As the name itself indicates, the entry and exit of Calcium ions are regulated by voltage or electricity. Upon exposure to high EMF, the Calcium channels or gates remain open for a longer duration than usual. This makes the Calcium ions on the outside, which are in higher concentration, flood into the cells. Because of this, the mitochondria i.e. powerhouse of the cells are not able to release Adenosine Triphosphate (ATP), which is a source of energy, thus making you feel tired, lethargic, weak, or in a state of confusion. This gradually will manifest into chronic diseases like heart disease, cancer, etc. You can refer to the following research paper for in-depth knowledge:

> ## EMF exposure increases calcium levels inside the cells
>
> "Electromagnetic Field Effects on Cells of the Immune System: The Role of Calcium Signaling." Walleczek J. FASEB Journal. Vol. 6, no. 13. (1992): 3177-85. doi: 10.1096/ fasebj.6.13.1397839.

Till this point we understood that we are fighting against two enemies, one being the side effects of the COVID Vaccine and the second being the invisible enemy –EMF, attacking us continuously without us being aware of it and killing us silently.

Now take a look at this link:

> ## emf-portal.org

This is your homework. If you visit this portal you will find more than 30,000 research papers substantiating the facts that I have presented in this chapter. Your work is to go through these research papers for more understanding of this looming invisible death threat.

Until now you were ignorant about this invisible threat as you are used to accessing information through social media only and no one bothers to dig deep into journals and research papers for a deeper understanding of the existing problem. Now that you know about it, you will need to do your own research. Closing your eyes does not mean the danger is not there or because it is invisible does not mean it is not dangerous.

Let me demonstrate this danger through this instrument called EMF Meter.

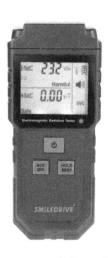

If you bring a switched-off mobile phone and turn on the EMF meter, it will display the radiation levels as negligible or zero. Now switch on the mobile, and you can see that the readings on the EMF meter start going up, but stay within safe levels. Now plug the charger into the mobile phone. The EMF meter will start beeping once you place it near the charging mobile. The beeping sound and the high readings show the radiations being emitted as extremely harmful.

Now there is homework for you. With the help of an EMF meter find out the radiations levels under the following conditions:

1. Radiation levels while using a mobile phone in a moving car.

2. Radiation levels in a parked car.

3.   Radiation levels of a charging mobile phone.

You will observe that the EMF radiation levels are higher when the car is moving at a higher speed. You will also observe that mobile phone radiations are higher when you are inside the car while it is parked than outside in the open. Mobile phones emit highly harmful radiation when they are getting charged.

To avoid exposure to such harmful radiation, you can charge the mobile away from your bedroom or where you are sitting. Switch off all lights and plug out all the gadgets from the electrical sockets. Avoid using mobile phones in moving vehicles. Doing so, you will realize that in the morning you wake up fresh and stay energized the entire day.

- **Avoid using cell phone in a moving car**
- **Avoid using cellphone in a parked car**
- **Never sleep with cellphone beside your bed side**

This is the first step towards reducing the burden of unnecessary exposure to EMF on your body.

In the next chapter, I will explain the solution or how we can shield ourselves from two deadly enemies i.e. a side effect of the COVID Vaccine and invisible EMF radiation.

CHAPTER -3

The Zero Volt Therapy

(This chapter is taken from the lecture of "Zero Volt Therapy" certification course).

In this chapter, you are going to learn one of the cheapest ways to heal with the least effort, getting the maximum benefit. You will learn a special technique. Once you learn it, you will understand that all kinds of pills that we humans are dependent upon most of the time, such as antidepressants, sleeping pills, painkillers, or say drugs we take to reduce blood pressure and blood sugar, or medicines we take to control heart diseases, and so on, will not be required. These medicines will no longer be needed if someone who is addicted to them learns this technique.

It's a very promising technique, called **'Zero Volt Therapy'**.

It is important to understand what Zero Volt Therapy is and how to use it.

It's the cheapest therapy and, in fact, it's free. Once you learn it, you can apply it throughout your life. You won't need any money. It gives you a free supply of medicine throughout your life.

To help you understand this, I will start by citing a very good example from China. In 1975, the city of Haicheng was hit by a major earthquake. Thankfully, only 2,000 people died even though the city had millions of residents. How did that happen? Local authorities took a timely decision to evacuate the residents based on unusual behavior detected among animals in Haicheng a few days before the quake struck. Since the authorities moved almost the entire human population outside the zone, fewer deaths happened. It is well known that animals can predict such events and disasters days before they happen.

Now, let us look at another example, also from China. It's also about an earthquake that happened in Tangshan in 1976. Here also, unusual behavior of animals and birds could be seen. So, the local authorities consulted earth scientists called seismologists and asked them to come and carry out a survey to decide whether to evacuate people or whether it was safe for the residents to remain there.

The seismologists surveyed and concluded that no earthquake was expected in the region. They themselves also decided to stay in Tangshan for another night. Next day, a major earthquake occurred and about 2,40,000 people died. The seismologists were also among those who died.

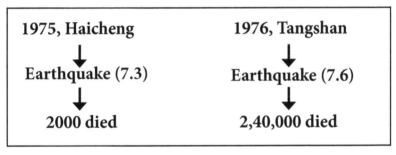

The point is that humans cannot predict natural disasters, but animals can. All other animals, including birds and even insects, can sense whenever a tsunami or earthquake is about to happen. When such quakes take place, notice that humans die and so do animals that are trapped. But the rest of the animals leave and survive the disaster.

It is important to note here that there is something called the sixth sense that animals and birds have – it is something that humans don't have.

I am emphasizing all this because it's eventually related to Zero Volt Therapy that I will go into detail later.

You might have seen some videos or read books, about how animals show unusual behavior before an earthquake strikes. I have also compiled a video of such behavior which can be seen on this link: www.biswaroop.com/zvtbook. These videos clearly indicate that animals can sense that a disaster is about to happen. Much research on this subject is being done all over the world to prove this observation right.

In fact, there's very good research on the unusual behavior of ants, which was carried out for three years. It found that ants change their direction much before, often months in advance, before an earthquake strikes.

Early Results of Three-Year Monitoring of Red Wood Ants' Behavioral Changes and Their Possible Correlation with Earthquake Events. Animals (Basel).

Berberich G, Berberich M, Grumpe A, Wöhler C, Schreiber U. 2013 Feb 4;3(1):63-84. doi: 10.3390/ani3010063. PMID: 26487310; PMCID: PMC4495521.

Similarly, there is another research paper on the behaviour of animals and other living organisms before earthquakes.

Nature of Pre-Earthquake Phenomena and their Effects on Living Organisms. Animals (Basel).

Freund F, Stolc V. 2013 Jun 6;3(2):513-31. doi: 10.3390/ani3020513. PMID: 26487415; PMCID: PMC4494396.

Then there's this other research paper in which the authors came close to finding the cause or reason behind how animals can sense a coming earthquake. That reason has to do with the earth's electric field. This is where you will get the first major clue. That clue is – humans are the only animals who wear shoes.

We, humans, are the only ones to remain insulated from the earth. We are not directly connected to the earth, whereas all animals are directly connected to the earth, all the time. Even birds are connected to the earth because they often sit on the branches of trees, which are conductive.

Much before earthquakes happen, possibly months, some kind of electromagnetic changes happen in the earth's core. One can feel electromagnetic changes if one is constantly in direct contact with the earth.

We humans, if such electromagnetic changes happen, will not be able to feel that because we are constantly insulated from the earth. All other animals will be able to feel that. It is because of this, animals run for their safety before natural disasters happen, and most of the time, they manage to save themselves.

Earth electric field negative anomalies as earthquake pre-cursors

Sergey Smirnov, Institute of Cosmophysical Researches and Radio Wave Propagation FEB RAS, Paratunka, Kamchatsky Kray, Russia

---

Here, we have to understand that the human body is also an electrical body. As I explained to you in the last chapter, all living beings also have electrical fields. When a doctor uses a stethoscope on a patient, what he's trying to hear is the cardiac electrical signal. Also, through ECG and EEG, we try to check the electrical signal. When a person dies, which is what we call cardiac arrest, what doctors sometimes do is, they try to give a shock or electric current to revive him.

So, electric current is more important than even oxygen. Without oxygen, you can survive for four to five minutes. But without an electrical signal, you cannot survive even for four to five seconds. So, an electrical signal is more important for humans to survive than even oxygen.

If we can restore this electrical signal, or if we can restore our conductivity with the earth, maybe there will be a possibility we can heal ourselves better. We have tried this out on many patients, and we got extraordinary results.

That's why I thought of sharing this technique with you through this book on Zero Volt Therapy.

We did a study on thalassemia patients. We took on board about 100 children with thalassemia. In thalassemia, the patient needs a blood transfusion almost every week, every two weeks, or at least once every month. Parents are told that they need to transfuse blood into their children, who have thalassemia, for their entire lifetime.

But we helped these children get two to three hours of contact with earth every day, along with some other changes, and we got extraordinary results. If you want to know about those results and their stories, you can read the book "Cure For Blood Disorders". You can get it on www.biswaroop.com/ebook.

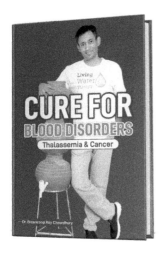

Let me now tell you how we helped children with thalassemia come out of the vicious cycle of blood transfusion. We did it by balancing the three factors of life – something we call the **'circadian triangle'**.

This we learned in the last chapter also.

One factor is, we have to understand that we are all chemical beings. In the last two years, those who attended my medical nutrition class learned how to regain chemical balance through DIP Diet and 3 Step Flu Diet. This comprises hormonal balance, nutrition balance, and vitamin and minerals balance. So, by changing your lifestyle and changing your food habits, you can restore chemical balance, and once you achieve that, you can get rid of diseases.

The second factor is called *physical balance*. It's got to do with the balance of your body, your bones, your structure, your skin, etc. To balance that, we learned through emergency and pain management online training, especially things like hot water immersion and heat protocol, that we can achieve a physical balance for our bodies.

The third factor is called electrical balance. This dimension was missing from our lives earlier on. Once we can establish the *electrical balance* as well, with the other two, my experience says you can resolve all kinds of illnesses. Once you establish balance across all three factors, you can achieve circadian rhythm, which is the biological clock of the body

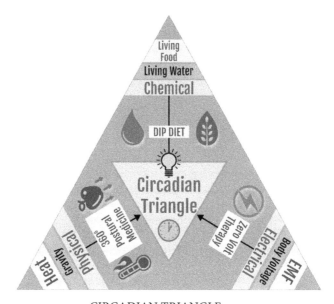

CIRCADIAN TRIANGLE

So, what we have been missing out on so far is the electrical balance in the bodies of the children with thalassemia. How do you restore electrical balance in them? Simply by encouraging them to be directly in contact with the Earth. Have a look at these interesting photographs to know how we did that.

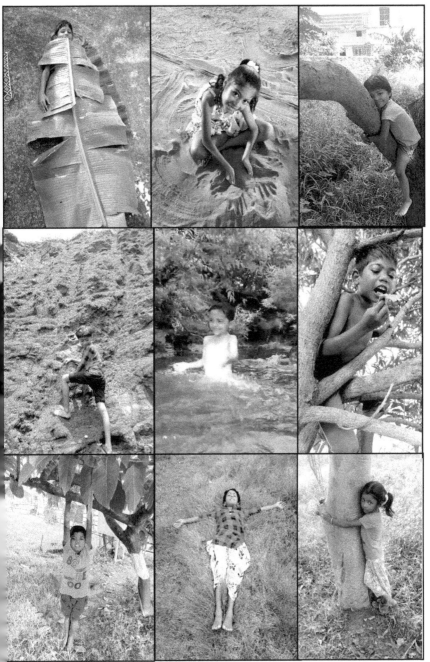

VARIOUS GROUNDING/EARTHING TECHNIQUES

You can see that they got connected with the Earth directly through recreational activities. When you touch the branch of the tree, even then you are connected to the Earth. Also, when you are in the river or in a pond, you are directly connected to the ground. If you do that for two to three hours daily, preferably for six hours, you can accelerate the healing process.

So, what exactly happens when you are directly touching the Earth? Remember, when you walk on the ground bare feet, each foot has about 1,400 nerves, and those nerve endings are directly touching the Earth. So, the body starts receiving the electrons through those nerve endings under your feet, and the healing process accelerates.

Let's look at one very interesting research paper that says, 'once you are in contact with the ground, through the donation of electrons from the Earth, your blood viscosity becomes normal'. It's all about blood viscosity.

Grounding reduces RBC aggregation, increases the surface charge on it and reduces the blood viscosity

Chevalier G, Sinatra ST, Oschman JL, Delany RM. Earthing (grounding) the human body reduces blood viscosity-a major factor in cardiovascular disease. J Altern Complement Med. 2013 Feb;19(2):102-10. doi: 10.1089/acm.2011.0820. Epub 2012 Jul 3.

In the last few months, you have seen a lot of people dying suddenly. One of the causes of the sudden deaths is the effect of the Covid vaccine, as I told you in the previous chapter, and the cause is blood clots. If you want to avoid blood clotting, one of the easiest ways to do it is to remain in touch with the Earth.

Once you are in contact with the ground, the research paper says, it reduces the blood viscosity. The lower the blood viscosity, the lower is the blood clotting factor. The lower the blood clotting factor, the chances of cardiac arrest and heart arrest gets reduced.

Now, here is a very interesting article, and I recommend you read it. Also, there are many research papers on this subject showing that remaining in touch with the Earth helps you reverse disease and get protection from adversities.

One of those research papers is about the 'health implications of reconnecting the human body to the Earth's surface electrons'. This is something that you should read.

Earthing: Health Implications of Reconnecting the Human Body to the Earth's Surface Electrons

J Environ Public Health. 2012; 2012: 291541.

Yet another research was published in the Journal of Alternative and Complementary Medicine.

Earthing the Human Body Influences Physiologic Processes

The journal of alternative and complementary medicine volume 17, number 4, 2011, pp. 1–8

I collected all this research and I made a summary out of it. According to the summary, if you remain grounded every day of your life for a few hours, it will help you rapidly reduce inflammation, eliminate pain, get more energy, reduce stress, and get more sleep.

Here is the compilation of the conclusion of the various research papers on this subject.

- **Rapid reduction of inflammation**
- **Rapid reduction or elimination of chronic pain**
- **Better supply of vital oxygen & nutrition to the cells and tissues of the body**
- **Reduced stress**
- **Increased Energy**
- **Improved sleep**
- **Accelerated healing from injuries & surgery**

BENEFITS OF GROUNDING/EARTHING

You have understood a very important thing. That is, when you are grounded, you start getting cured. How remaining in touch with the Earth helps you, for that you have to understand one word, called 'inflammation'.

Inflammation is the first thing that happens just before you get a disease. It is the precursor to any disease. Whether it's heart disease, cancer, Alzheimer's, or metabolic syndrome, inflammation is the central character. Once you understand inflammation, it will be easy to understand everything else. So, let's first try to understand what inflammation is.

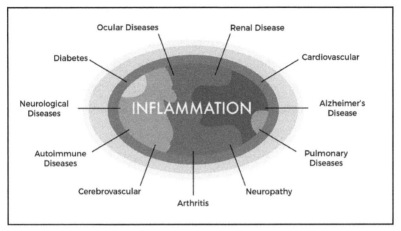

Inflammation is not a bad thing when it happens for a brief period of time. Actually, inflammation is your body's immune system response. It's like your body's security dog, for example. Let's say, you have a security dog. When robbers suddenly attack you, the security dog will take charge and chase the robbers away by biting them or by barking at them.

That is the essential purpose of a security dog. But if the security dog continues to bark and bites harmless people including you, even after the robbers are gone, then it becomes a problem for you.

It is the same case with inflammation. Whenever your body is attacked by some pathogen, such as bacteria or virus, or if there's some injury from an accident, your immunity becomes active and as a result of that, some inflammatory response takes place. The primary goal of the response is to overcome the particular challenge.

But as it happens with many of us, when that challenge is gone, the inflammation keeps on growing and becomes a headache. Now if I ask you, how will you silence the security dog, you will feed the dog with meat or something that works, and maybe it will stop barking and biting.

Similarly, how to stop the inflammation? The free radicals have one unpaired electron. Now, if you feed electrons to the inflammation, then the inflammation will reduce, the free radicals will reduce, and as a result, the disease can be reversed.

Understand one thing, the earth is the biggest donor of electrons. When you get connected with the earth, you receive those electrons.

Through thunderstorms earth receives electrons and how you receive electrons from the earth, let us understand with the help of a simple demonstration. So, I have two glasses. Both are connected by a pipe.

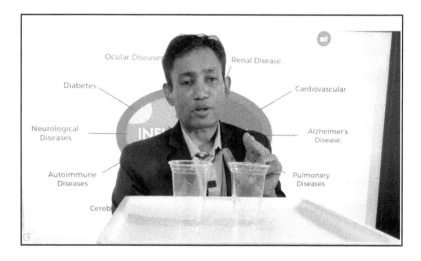

When I fill water into one glass, the water flows into the other glass till the water levels are the same.

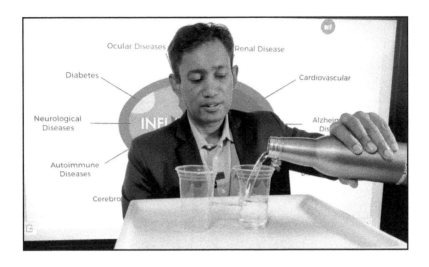

So, the water flows from the first glass to the second glass, that is, from the glass to my left to the one to my right. After a while, the flow stops because the water level is the same in both glasses.

Now, let's say, I fill some more water into the glass to my right.

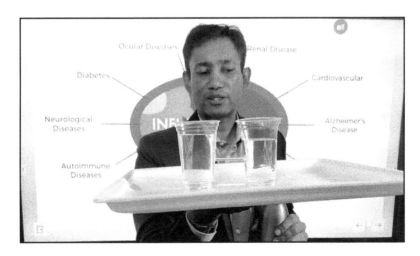

What happens is that the water flows in the reverse direction, and it continues to flow till the water levels are again in balance. So basically, the water flow takes place to balance or equalize the two water levels. Once the levels equalize, the water flow stops.

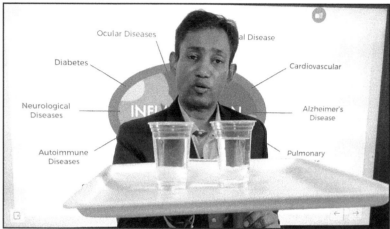

The same principle is at work if you ground yourself or when you directly touch the earth. At the time you touch the earth, your body is electron-deficient while the earth is full of electrons. The electrons start flowing into the body till the time the number of electrons in your body and the number of electrons in the earth is at the same level. We call that scenario 'zero volt'. The voltage of the earth is known to be zero. If you check your voltage with help of a voltmeter at that time you'll find that your body has zero volt.

When your body is not grounded or it is not connected to the earth for example while you are wearing shoes or are in an enclosed room; that time the voltmeter will show some reading on its display screen

But the body's healing can start only after the voltage comes down to zero. That can happen only if someone or something donates electrons to your body. The best source of electrons is the earth. So, if I touch the earth, electrons will start to freely flow into my body. Within the first 10 seconds, my body's voltage will become zero. That's when my body's inflammation will start to slowly disappear. Once the inflammation disappears, the disease in the body will also start to disappear gradually.

Essentially, this is the cheapest method by which you can heal yourself. Rather, it's a free method of doing so.

Ultimately, you need to remember that all serious diseases can be called 'chronic inflammation'. And the cause of chronic inflammation is 'electron deficiency'.

Chronic Inflammation = Electron deficiency

Till now, you have understood that by being in touch with the earth, just like other animals, we can resolve many health-related problems.

Now the question is, without having direct contact with the earth, how to still get connected with it? We live in city-centric conditions where we live in apartment buildings in which it may not be possible to remain grounded or remain in touch with the earth for long durations – say two to six hours a day.

Let's now look at what Richard Feynman, a Noble prize winner, once came up with. He gave us something that's called the 'Umbrella Effect of Earthing'.

Umbrella effect of Earthing

Richard Feynman
(Noble Prize Winner)

According to it, you don't need to go out in the open. You just take a copper wire, take one end of it, take it all the way outside, say from your apartment's window, take it straight to the ground, dig up the ground a little bit, and place one end of the copper wire into it.

The earth will start donating electrons through that copper wire straight to your body, and you will receive them in a manner as if you are directly in contact with the earth. This is what Feynman called the 'Umbrella Effect of Earthing'.

It's like this. If it's raining outside, you take out an umbrella. By taking out an umbrella, you cannot guarantee that you will not get wet at all. But you can guarantee that you will be less wet than you would be without an umbrella. You will get a sprinkle of rain on you despite using the umbrella, but overall, you will be protected from the rain. In the same manner, if you remain earthed through the copper wire, you will get most of the benefits.

So, we got that in 1964. But before him, in a book written in 1940, I found a reference to 'Grounding for Health'. The book is called Cosmo-Electro Culture for Land and Man. If you want to read the book, visit the link www.biswaroop.com/zvt.

You will find the mention of earthing for health benefits, in Ayurveda literature, written about 3000 years ago.

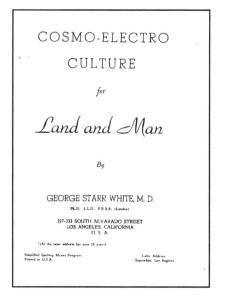

COSMO-ELECTRO
CULTURE

for

Land and Man

By

GEORGE STARR WHITE, M. D.
Ph.D. LL.D. F.R.S.A. (London)

327-333 SOUTH ALVARADO STREET
LOS ANGELES, CALIFORNIA
U. S. A.

(At the same address for over 35 years)

Simplified Spelling Means Progress.
Printed in U.S.A.

Cable Address
Starrwhite, Los Angeles

That was the time when we first realized that remaining in contact with the Earth protects us from various diseases. Not only that, but it can also help you reverse and cure diseases. It's not even necessary to directly touch the Earth. The benefits can be achieved through the conducting wire.

I demonstrated the same principle with the example of the two glasses I showed you earlier. If the two glasses are kept away from each other over a longer distance, all you would need is a longer pipe to connect the two, and the two water levels will remain the same.

Similarly, the human body, you and me, can be in contact with the earth even by being distant from it, simply by using a copper wire. So, this is called 'Zero Voltage Therapy'.

There have been many research papers on this subject on the benefits human beings get when they are connected to the earth. In one of those interesting papers, they designed a yoga mat and grounded it to the earth, after which they found benefits.

Richard Brown and Gaétan Chevalier, "Grounding the Human Body During Yoga Exercise with a Grounded Yoga Mat Reduces Blood Viscosity," Open Journal of Preventive Medicine 5 (2015): 159-168, doi: 10.4236/ojpm.2015.54019.

Here is one such yoga mat that we use at the HIIMS Premier Hospital in Gurgaon, India. Take a look at the picture on the next page, all the patients are sitting on the yoga mat and their bare feet are touching the mat. They are basically grounded or earthed even though they are inside the building.

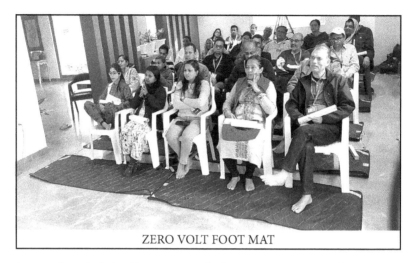

ZERO VOLT FOOT MAT

At our hospital itself, we noticed that patients reported receiving immense benefits. Over here, it's a regular feature for our patients to remain grounded for at least 12-14 hours a day, when they're having a training session, or even when they're sleeping, with their bed sheets connected directly to the earth.

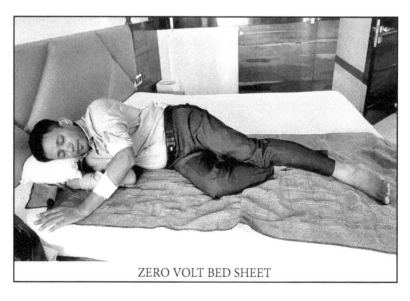

ZERO VOLT BED SHEET

Our hospital is not the only one in the world to be using Zero Volt Therapy to heal patients.

Before us, there have been several hospitals and research centers that used this technique to accelerate healing among patients.

A very important example to look at is the Tour de France cycling event. Like the Olympics, it's a prestigious, world-class cycling championship. It happens over a period of several days when the cyclists need to ride through different types of terrain throughout the day. In the process, they often fall from their cycles or meet with accidents, or injure and break their legs, etc.

The night, the cyclists halt in some hotel, and that is the only time they get, those few hours in the night, to heal themselves. In those few hours, to heal themselves very fast, in addition to all kinds of conventional first aid that's applied; they also use Zero Volt Therapy, getting connected to the ground through a conductive wire.

There's an interesting excerpt transcribed from a video (video is available at this link: www.biswaroop.com/zvtbook) that tells us how Zero Volt Therapy is used in world-class sports events and championships.

VIDEO TRANSCRIPTION :

Speaker 1: *"The earthing technology is essential to deliver earth's electrons to the body by direct skin contact with the help of product (earthing tool). Even though a rider may not be injured but the severe physical & mental strain needs to be discharged from the body while the rider is relaxing and recovering. So we use the earthing technology at night to make sure that they get up the next day fully recovered. The second use of the earthing technology is to accelerate tissue repair & wound healing from the injuries that may be sustained during the day in the 'tour de France'. The athletes reported & observed better sleep, less pain, more energy, and faster recovery from injury on a routine regular basis."*

Speaker 2: George Hincapie (Rider 'Tour de France' Discovery channel, Pro cycling team): *"The Earth technology works out great. It seems like we are sleeping in a lot better with this. My injury got a lot better after I got up the next morning using earthing technology specially putting patches directly on the injury."*

Speaker 1: *"Yaroslav Papowich crashed on a time-trial, and had massive abrasions on his right hip & right elbow. The moment we got back to the hotel, we used the earthing technology immediately to start to accelerate his recovery. He was able to get up & compete fully the following day &put in one of the most significant contributions to help in Alberto win that tour de France.*

When it gets really hot in France in July. The asphalt that the riders ride on starts to crack and blister and gets soft. If a rider falls on it it's like falling on a cheese grater. In one of the cases, Benjamin Thomas had been seriously injured. He received some of the deepest penetrating lacerations that I had ever seen. When we got back to the hotel, we put the earthing technology on him. He slept all night. He got up the next day and was able to compete and he was able to finish the tour.

The video tells us how athletes are healing themselves overnight using Zero Volt Therapy. So basically, when you are connecting yourself to the earth, your body's voltage becomes zero. And when it becomes zero, your body's healing process gets accelerated, whether it's an external injury or whether it's a disease.

There have been many research papers on this kind of strategy, or healing process, or treatment protocol. There have been many.

"One-Hour Contact with the Earth's Surface (Grounding) Improves Inflammation and Blood Flow-A Randomized, Double-Blind, Pilot Study," Gaétan Chevalier, G. Melvin, and T. Barsotti, Health 7 (2015): 1022-1059, doi: 10.4236/ health.2015.78119.

R. A. Passie et al., "Electrical Grounding Improves Vagal Tone in Preterm Infants," Neonatology 112 (2017): 187-192.

Karol Sokal and Pawel Sokal, "Earthing the Human Organism Influences ioelectrical Processes," Journal of Alternative and Complementary Medicine 18, no. 3 (2012): 229-234.

So, I collected all of them and made a summary of them. Let me share that summary with you. It's something we ourselves experienced with the patients in our hospital.

Zero Volt (Earth) Therapy

Time	Effect on body
10 Seconds	Your voltage will be zero
20 minutes	Improvement in mood/stress
30-45 minutes	Relief from palpitation
1 hour	Pain relief
1-2 hour	Better sleep
Overnight	Fast wound healing, less stiffness, Parkinson relief, reduction in B.P.
7 days	Reduced B.P. (for diabetes patients)
1 month	Blood disorder reversal

So, when you ground yourself even with an electric wire, within the first 10 seconds, your body's voltage becomes zero. Then within the first 20 minutes, your stress reduces, and your mood refreshes. Within 30-45 minutes, palpitations go down and you become normal.

Within one hour, patients report clear-cut pain relief, such as relief from knee-joint pain, back pain, headache, etc. Within one to two hours, they go into a state of deep sleep; especially those patients who otherwise had problems sleeping.

If people sleep overnight on zero-volt bed sheets, those with Parkinson's disease will see a reduction in symptoms, and they will see relief in terms of blood pressure and stiffness of the body. They will see relief in terms of wound healing as well.

Within seven days of using zero-volt bed sheets, most patients see a reduction in BP, and blood sugar, eventually helping taper down the use of drugs. Within one month of use, we have seen patients experience a reversal of blood disorder, such as with thalassemia patients.

With those patients, we started the zero voltage treatment protocol in July and now this is December. So, in this span of six months, they didn't need a blood transfusion, they are able to maintain their hemoglobin levels, maintain their energy levels, and they are as normal and healthy as any other person. That is the power of Zero Volt Therapy.

Now I will explain to you how to use Zero Volt Therapy at home step by step.

First, you need to check the voltage of your body. To check it, you will have to use a voltmeter. In a volt meter, there are two terminals. Put the black terminal in 'COM', and then place the red one in the other terminal.

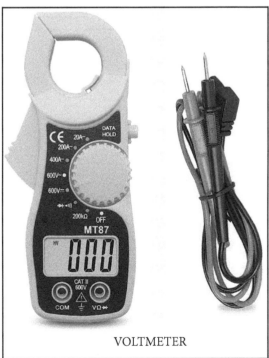

VOLTMETER

Next, you will have to switch it on. Since we are interested in checking the voltage, put the voltage mode on.

Whenever you need to check the voltage of your body, you will have to touch the red terminal. Or, if you want to check the voltage of anything, the object has to be in contact with the red terminal. The other one, which is the black one, always needs to be connected to the Earth.

How can you connect it to the earth? One way to do it is to connect it to the grounding hole (or earthing hole) of an electrical socket in your home. Once you connect it to the grounding/ earthing hole of the socket, the volt meter will start to show the voltage. That is your body's voltage.

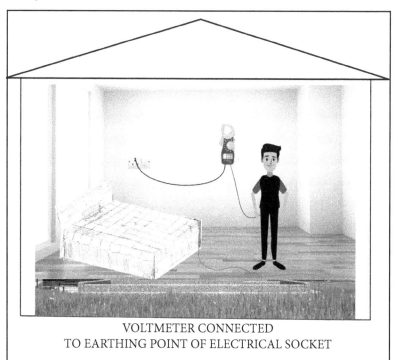

VOLTMETER CONNECTED
TO EARTHING POINT OF ELECTRICAL SOCKET

But the problem is, here in India; in most of the houses - even at my place and my office– the earthing is not proper. In some places, the earthing is not in place at all.

So generally, the top hole of a socket is not in working condition. If you are not sure whether the socket hole of your home is in working condition or not, connect the black wire directly to the earth.

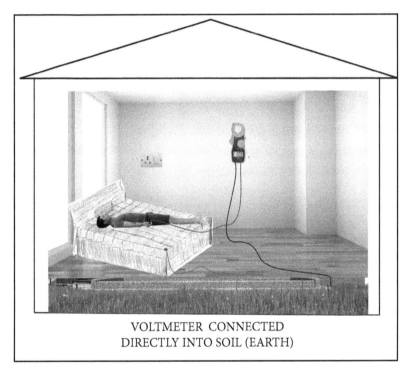

VOLTMETER CONNECTED
DIRECTLY INTO SOIL (EARTH)

So whenever you want to check your body's voltage, ensure that you wear shoes and don't directly be in touch with the earth. Now hold the red terminal of the voltmeter making it touch your bare skin, while the black terminal is connected to the Earth. To connect to the earth, either you should directly connect the wire to the ground through an extension cord, or simply connect it directly if you are outdoors. But don't forget to wear shoes. Also, you can use the socket, if it is working.

Now, I will tell you about the Zero Volt Therapy bed sheet. On this bed sheet, there are multiple threads. These threads are made of copper and they are 1mm thick. Each thread is made of 16 finer threads, making it 1mm thick.

Along with that, you will also get this extension wire that is 10 meters long. So, even if you reside on the second floor of a building, this wire can be connected to the ground through your window. This is a copper wire with 32 threads and a thickness of 1.5mm. It has a copper rod (1 foot long). It goes directly into the earth.

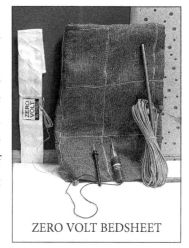

ZERO VOLT BEDSHEET

Now spread the bedsheet on your bed. Connect any one corner of the bedsheet with the extension copper wire with the help of connectors on the corner of the bedsheet and one end of the copper wire. Put the other end of the extension copper wire with copper rod directly 1 foot deep into the soil. Now you are all set to receive electrons.

The process happens as you touch the bed sheet with bare hands or feet, or when you sleep on it.

Also, when you sleep on it, you will have to ensure that you wear minimum clothes, so that much of your body touches the wire. And while in a sleeping position, you can check the real voltage of your body at that moment. After sleeping on this bedsheet, your body's voltage will come to zero in about 10 seconds. If it comes to zero, it would mean the arrangements have been done properly.

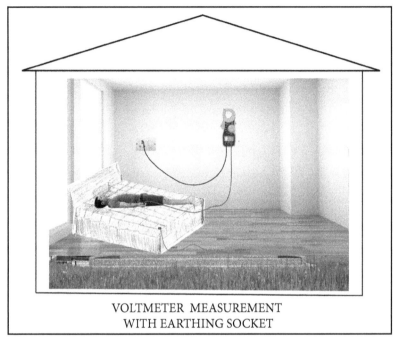

VOLTMETER MEASUREMENT
WITH EARTHING SOCKET

So, now you know how to check your voltage when you are not grounded, and also when you are in contact with the earth through this bed sheet. Once you have checked your voltage, you can remove the voltmeter. Now, if the socket is not working, or if your building is not grounded properly, in that case, you will have to directly connect with the earth. That way, too, you can get the right voltage, which is expected to be zero, if you are sleeping or lying down on this zero-volt bed sheet.

This is the complete set to help you install the zero-volt bed sheet properly, and to ensure that you are receiving electrons from the Earth. It will also help you understand what your voltage was before, and what it was later on.

Once the voltage comes down to zero, then it is confirmed that the setting has been done properly.

When you use this bed sheet, you will have to check the continuity of the electron flow. To check it, I have provided a continuity tester.

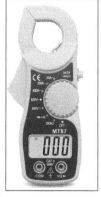

To check the continuity, touch one of the terminals of the continuity tester with any of the wires on the zero-volt bed sheet, and the other terminal of the continuity tester with wires anywhere on the bedsheet. The moment you touch it, the red light will blink. This will be proof that your zero-volt bed sheet is conductive and all the wires are in continuity and the circuit is not broken. This test can be repeated by touching other wires on the bed sheet. If every time the light blinks it confirms that the bed sheet is conductive.

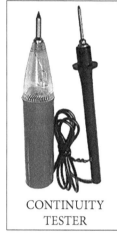

CONTINUITY TESTER

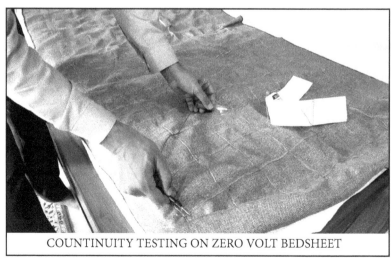

COUNTINUITY TESTING ON ZERO VOLT BEDSHEET

But in the market, some people are selling zero-volt bed sheets claiming that they are conductive; they look quite like this one. But they are poor conductor. Their conductivity can be tested with the help of this continuity tester.

If it is a good conductor, the light will blink. But if the light is not blinking. That means it is a poor conductor. It may be conducting electrons, but overall it's a very poor conductor. So poor that the light doesn't blink. This means it has failed the continuity test. So, avoid buying such bed sheets.

When you are using the zero-volt bed sheets for a long time, the wire may break in between and it may not be conducive anymore. So, you need to check and recheck your zero-volt bed sheets properly from time to time using a continuity meter. To help you understand it in a better way you can visit this link and watch the video (Continuity Meter Test) available on this link: www.biswaroop.com/zvtbook

This link also has a video, where I explained Zero Volt Therapy in detail during one of my lectures on Naturopathy day.

Similarly another video from Vietnam in which you will find me explaining the same science to a group of patients and students. Watch this as it will help you understand the concept better.

Watching these videos will clarify things more clearly. You can install the bed sheets properly without any mistakes and check them with the help of a continuity tester.

Another very important Video on 'How to Check Earthing of Your Home'?

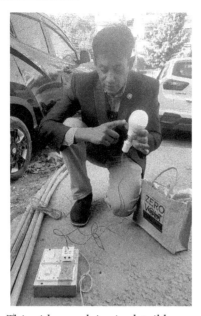 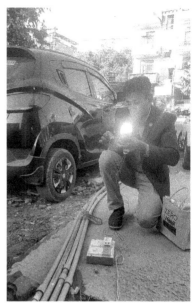

This video explains in detail how you can check if the electrical wiring and sockets at your home are properly earthed or not. Whether your building's earthing is proper or not, or whether you have correctly grounded the bed sheet or not? Through this series of videos, you will understand how to use it properly. My observation is that when patients use it, or when they come to our hospital, 80% of them report good sleep, almost 75% report reduced pain, and nearly 100% of them report some kind of benefit.

There is yet another video from Switzerland of my friend Nigel Kingsley who has also installed a Zero Volt Bedsheet at his home and reaping its benefit.

So, with this, I end this chapter hoping you will charge your body with 'Zero Volt Bedsheet' and get up every day fully energized and refreshed free from any kind of pain and stay healthy.

For all the videos in this chapter visit this link :
www.biswaroop.com/zvtbook

SECTION -II

Key Outcomes of Cure@72 hrs: Observational study

What will happen during the first 72 hours, while we try to bring back the chemical, physical and electrical balance, by trying to correct the body clock?

In this section, I share the summary of the observational study done through the collaborative efforts of Shridhar University, Pilani, Rajasthan & Dayanand Ayurvedic College, Jalandhar. The study was done on our recently concluded Cure @ 72 hrs program at HIIMS Premier Hospital, Gurugram.

The key guidelines maintained during the 72hrs stay of the patients are:-

1) Patients were encouraged to sleep in accordance with their age, as per the table given below.

Age	Ideal	Not recommended	Normal	Borderline	Abnormal	Normal	Borderline	Abnormal
0-3 months	14-17	<11 or >19	0-30 min	30-45 min	>45 min	Normal to wake up a few times		
4-11 months	12-15	<10 or >18	0-30 min	30-45 min	>45 min	Normal to wake up a few times		
1-2 years	11-14	<9 or >17	0-30 min	30-45 min	>45 min	1	2-3	>4
3-5 years	10-13	<8 or >16	0-30 min	30-45 min	>45 min	1	2-3	>4
6-13 years	9-11	<7 or >15	0-30 min	30-45 min	>45 min	1	2-3	>4
14-17 years	8-10	<7 or >13	0-30 min	30-45 min	>45 min	1	2	>3
18-25 years	7-9	<6 or >11	0-30 min	30-45 min	>45 min	1	2-3	>4
26-64 years	7-9	<6 or >10	0-30 min	30-45 min	>45 min	1	2-3	>4
>65 years	7-8	<6 or >10	0-30 min	30-60 min	>60 min	2	3	>4

2) We tried to maintain zero voltage of the patients, at least 10hrs per day. This was achieved by placing a zero volt bed sheet in their rooms and a zero-volt foot-mat in the training room under the chair of each participant.

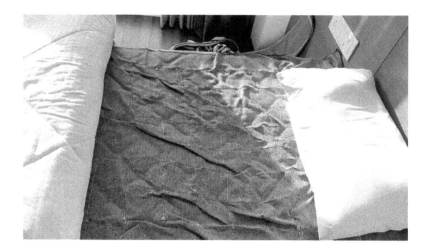

ZERO VOLT BEDSHEET IN ROOMS

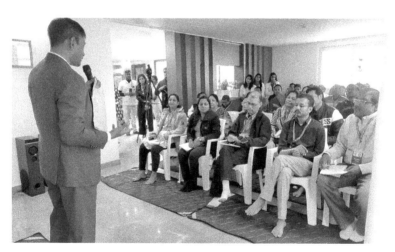

ZERO VOLT FOOT MATS IN TRAINING ROOM

3) Food in accordance with the DIP diet was provided during the entire stay.

4) Living water was provided from a 2-pot / 3-pot water system during the entire stay. To know more about it, read my book "The Cure for blood disorders".

5) To achieve physical balance, based on their symptoms (swelling, pain etc), patients were given specific therapies like hot water immersion, head down tilt, heat protocol or panchakarma, etc.

6) Patients were encouraged to get at least 10,000 lux -of light for more than 30 minutes during the first half of the day and were also asked to avoid the light of more than 50 lux at least 2 hours before sleep.

7) Patients were served food within the bracket of 11 hours ie between 8.00 am to 7:00 pm. For a time between 7:00 pm and to next day 8:00 am, they are asked to avoid eating. Drinking water was allowed without any restrictions.

8) CBC reports of the patients were taken at the beginning and the end of the 72 hours of camp. Other vitals like blood sugar, blood pressure, body weight, pain intensity, and energy level were collected several times per day during their entire stay in the hospital. Blood sugar sensors were implanted in the arms of 8 diabetes patients.

9) Drugs were tapered in accordance with the improvement of various parameters.

Observational study

Dr. Anu Bhardwaj (BAMS)
Dr. Namita Gupta (MBBS, MD)
Shridhar University- Rajasthan

Dr Aman Sanger (BAMS, MD)
Dayanand Ayurvedic College,
Jalandhar

The key outcome in 72 hours residential camp

1. 10 patients were taking antihypertensive medication at the time of joining the72 hours camp. By the end of the camp, about 70% of them could reduce their systolic blood pressure by an average of 20 mmHg.

2. Among the hypertension patients, 50% of them could taper down their drugs to zero.

3. 8 patients were on anti-diabetes medication. 62.5 % of them could taper their drugs by an average of 50%. 30% of patients could get rid of drugs completely.

4. 2 patients were insulin dependent. One patient could free himself completely from insulin. The other (type I) patient could reduce the dependency on insulin by 50%.

5. 8 patients reported constipation at the beginning of 72 hours program. 75% of them reported 100 % relief at the end of the program.

6. 12 patients were overweight(BMI >25). 75% could reduce their weight by an average of 1 kg.

7. 15 Patients reported pain (joint/back etc) at the beginning of 72 hours program. 80% got more than 50% relief by the end of the program.

8. Among the anemic patients, after 10 days of completing the 72 hours camp, the average increase in hemoglobin, Red blood cells

& packed cell volume were 0.3 gm/dl, 0.105 cell/MCL and 2.36% respectively. The highest increase in hemoglobin RBC count & PCV are 1.9 g/dl, 0.34 cell/MCL & 10.2% respectively (among the patients, who submitted their CBC reports).

Noticeable feedback

1. Rohit Chaudhary type 1 Diabetic patient, on day 2, his sugar level came down to 250 mg/dl from 600 mg/dl in an hour just by taking HWI and without insulin.

2. Sumit Arora had an amazing experience with matrabasti. He had immediate relief from chronic constipation. Further, he is reported to have discontinued the dependency on inhalers by the 3rd day of the camp.

3. Patient Shalini Prakash reported complete relief from severe knee pain within the first night of zero-volt bed sheet sleeping.

4. Mukesh Pahwa, from Australia who was suffering from swollen feet after 2 stents were implanted in June 2022, got rid of his swelling completely after LLHWI& banana therapy.

5. Renu Agarwal, came with the symptom of a spinning head & low energy. By the 3rd day, she got relief from both problems.

6. Pratyush Sarkar could reduce the dependency on drugs for the management of the pain of Fibromyalgia by 70% with noticeable relief in pain.

Goodwill Ambassador of "Zero Volt Therapy"

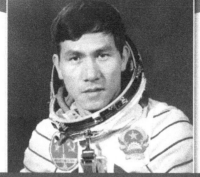

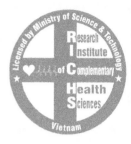

Lieutenant General Pham Tuan, the first Asian to fly to space

It's my priviledge, to be known to legendary Leutinent General Pham Tuan, who accepted our invitation and participated in our annual India Book of Records event on 11 September, 2022 in New Delhi, India.

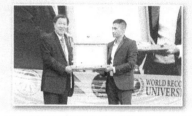

Again I got an opportunity to meet him exactly at the time when Vietnam was preparing to celebrate his completion of 50 years of Christmas Bombing (18-27 to Dec 1972), his major contribution in Vietnam war.

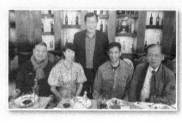

As he was convinced, that the **"Zero Volt Therapy"** will help the humanity in reducing pain, I received the following letter from him.

Dr. Biswaroop Roy Chowdhury

Ngày 21 tháng 12 năm 2022

Kính gửi Trung tướng Phạm Tuân,

Thật là một sự vinh hạnh khi được gặp ông vào tuần trước. Qua bức thư này, tôi muốn chia sẻ về công việc của mình tại RICHS* , một viện nghiên cứu trực thuộc IW Hội Kỷ lục Việt Nam và Tổ chức Kỷ lục châu Á hoạt động ở Ấn Độ và Việt Nam. Chúng tôi đang thúc đẩy khai niệm duy trì kết nối giữa con người với Trái đất vì lợi ích sức khỏe. Khái niệm này mang ý nghĩa là khám phá sự liên kết và tiếp xúc của cơ thể con người với diện tích tự nhiên của Trái đất vì những ích lợi sức khỏe. Ông là một vị Anh hùng Dân tộc Việt Nam, Anh hùng Liên bang Xô Viết, một nhân vật nổi tiếng mang tầm quốc tế và là 1 kỷ lục gia châu Á - người châu Á đầu tiên bay vào vũ trụ. Chúng tôi tin chắc rằng, nếu khái niệm này được phổ biến tử ông, mọi người sẽ nghiêm túc nhìn nhận và đón nhận nó hơn và cuối cùng thông điệp này sẽ thành công giúp nhân loại khỏe mạnh và bình yên hơn:

"Hãy kết nối với Trái đất vì sức khỏe thể chất và tinh thần của bạn"

Chúng tôi muốn mời ông trở thành đại sứ tinh thần trong dự án này.

Trân trọng cảm ơn ông

Tiến sĩ Biswaroop Roy Chowdhury Tổng Giám Đốc Tổ chức Kỷ lục châu Á.

* Research Institute of Complimentary Health Sciences (RICHS)

Kỷ lục gia châu Á

Kỷ lục gia Phạm Tuân

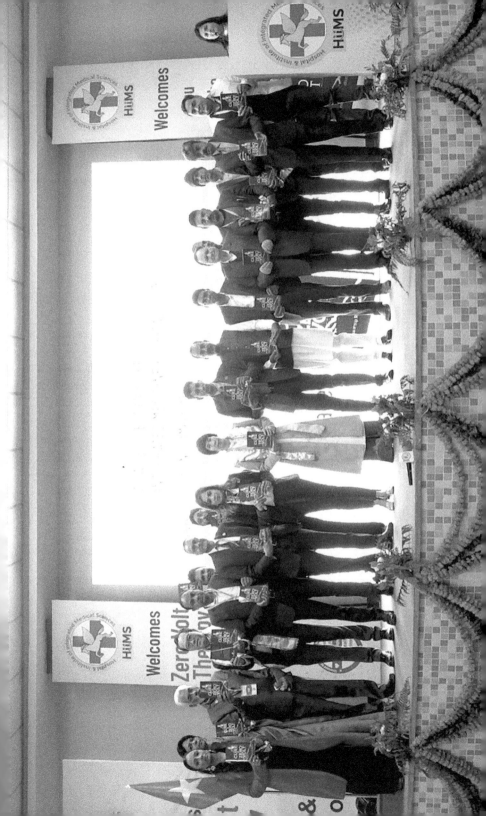

Books by Dr. Biswaroop Roy Chowdhury

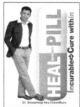

Price: ₹ 250/-
(Courier charges extra)

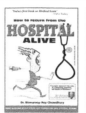

Price: ₹ 95/-
(Courier charges extra)

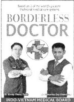

Price: ₹ 150/-
(Courier charges extra)

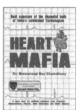

Price: ₹ 150/-
(Courier charges extra)

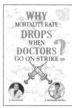

Price: ₹200/-
(Courier charges extra)

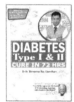

Price: ₹150/-
(Courier charges extra)

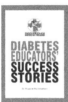

Price: ₹ 195/-
(Couner charges extra)

Price: ₹ 350/-
(Courier charges extra)

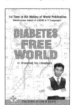

Price: ₹ 100/-
(Courier charges extra)

Price: ₹ 100/-
(Courier charges extra)

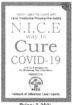

Price: ₹ 250/-
(Courier charges extra)

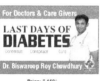

Price: ₹ 150/-
(Courier charges extra)

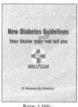

Price: ₹ 100/-
(Courier charges extra)

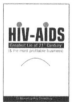

Price: ₹ 100/-
(Courier charges extra)

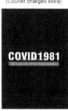

Price: ₹ 175/-
(Courier charges extra)

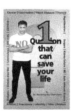

Price: ₹ 175/-
(Courier charges extra)

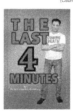

Price: ₹ 150/-
(Courier charges extra)

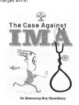

Price: ₹ 150/-
(Courier charges extra)

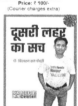

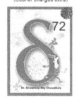

Price: ₹150/-
(Courier charges extra)

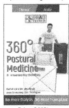

Price: ₹ 225/-
(Courier charges extra)

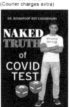

Price: ₹ 200/-
(Courier charges extra)

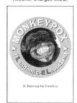

Price: ₹ 100/-
(Courier charges extra)

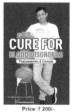

Price: ₹ 200/-
(Courier charges extra)

Buy online at: www.biswaroop.com/shop
Dynamic Memory Pvt. Ltd.
B-121, 2nd Floor, Green Fields, Faridabad-121010 (Haryana), Mob.:+91-9312286540
E-mail:biswaroop@biswaroop.com
(Available in Hindi/English, in all leading onlinestores)

Read/Subscribe
Fortnightly
Digital Magazine

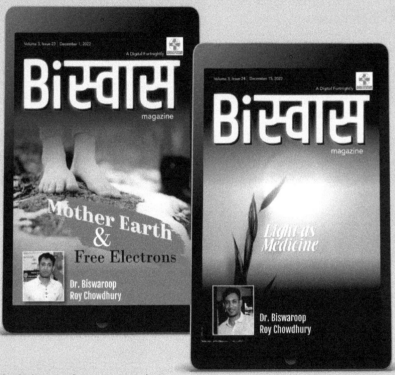

Chief Editor: Prof. Ainapur Purushottam

To read, go to:
www.biswaroop.com/biswas

You don't need medication, you just need education

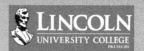

3 Months Online Certification
on
Advance Nutrition Therapy
from
Lincoln University College, Malaysia

Overview: From common cold to Cancer, from headache to heart attack, you can be your own healer. This training comes with a unique tool kit packed with 28 ingredients, the right combination of it can work as a medicine for more than 60 kinds of common illnesses. This training will empower you with skills to heal and will make you realize that your home is the best place to reclaim your health.

Duration: 3 Months

Content:
- Diagnosis of Lifestyle Illness
- Diagnosis of Infectious Diseases
- Food –Medicine Interaction
- Mechanism of Medicine in Body
- Mechanism of Food in Body
- When the Food is Medicine
- When Medicine is Poison
- Common Kitchen Herbs and their Medicinal Usages
- Timeline of Recovery of Common Illnesses
- Food Calculation for Overall Nutrition
  Plants V/S Animal Food

Take-Home Material :
- Hospital in a Box
- Game of Life Chart
- Snake Ladder Nutrition Game
- Reference Book

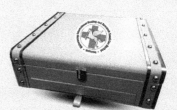

Course Fee: **INR 21,000/- (including GST + Courier)**
Mode of Training: **Online/ viva (oral examination) through a video call**

To register go to www.biswaroop.com/mn

CALL US :+91-9312286540 MAIL US: biswaroop@biswaroop.com

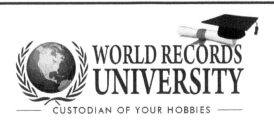

WORLD RECORDS UNIVERSITY

—— CUSTODIAN OF YOUR HOBBIES ——

The World Records University is an autonomous university formed by the conglomeration of 'Record Books' around the world. Its associates include Asia Book of Records, Vietnam Book of Records, Indo-China Book of Records, India Book of Records, Nepal Book of Records, World Records Union, World Creativity Science Academy, and Indo-Vietnam Medical Board. It has its registered Offices in UK, US, India and Vietnam

Steps for applying for the Honorary Doctorate Degree:

Step 1: Request application form at info@worldrecordsuniversity.com. Submit the Honorary Doctorate Degree application form along with a scanned copy of your record certificate to info@worldrecordsuniversity.com

Step 2: Your application will undergo preliminary scrutiny for approval.

Step 3: After approval /acceptance of the application, you will be required to deposit the processing fee.

Step 4: Prepare a thesis of your record breaking journey in accordance with the format of World Records University (to be sent to you).

Step 5: World Records University will scrutinize and provide you with feedback on your thesis.

Step 6: After making changes as suggested by the feedback, you will have to submit a hard copy of the thesis. An expert panel will accept and approve the thesis. On approval you will receive a confirmation email for your Honorary Doctorate Degree.

Step 7: You will receive your Honorary Doctorate Degree at the Global Convocation to be held in India or abroad.

Step 8: Submit the soft copy of the thesis to info@worldrecordsuniversity.com.

CONTACT:
Phone: +91-9555008451
Email: info@worldrecordsuniversity.com
Webiste: www.worldrecordsuniversity.co.uk

Certification Partner

The Ultimate honor for the record holders

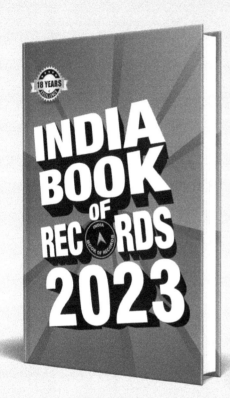
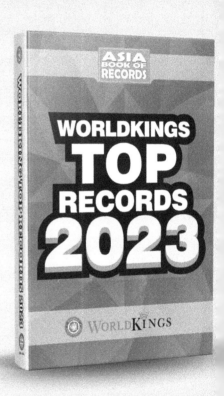
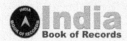

Health Freedom
with
N.I.C.E & W.I.S.E

Dr. Biswaroop Roy Chowdhury and his N.I.C.E (Network of Influenza Care Experts) team have helped and cured more than 50,000 COVID-19 and other infectious/communicable diseases patients (including smallpox, typhoid, tuberculosis) with zero medicine / money / mortality.

Now health freedom through W.I.S.E (Wellness and Inflammatory Syndrome Experts) for more than 60 types of non-communicable / lifestyle illnesses.

Service to the Nation in 2 Steps

Step-1: Call our 24x7 helpline number: +91-8587059169.

Step-2: Fill the details of the patient in the link given below.

www.biswaroop.com/nice
(Influenza/Communicable diseases)

www.biswaroop.com/wise
(Lifestyle/Non-communicable diseases)

Let every morning be the Hunza Morning

If you have decided to pick only one of my suggestions for the sake of your health, then take this suggestion :

Stop consuming tea specially, morning tea. The early morning tea makes the inner lining of your intestinal wall acidic, as after a long night of fasting your stomach is empty and craving for food. An acidic stomach on a regular basis is the single biggest cause of all kind of inflammatory and lifestyle diseases including arthritis, Diabetes etc.

How to stop craving of tea ⟶ Switch to Hunza Tea

Hunza Civilization: Hunza people are the Indians living at extreme northwest of India in Hindu Kush range. They are known to be one of the world's healthiest civilizations, often living up to the age of 110 years.

How to prepare Hunza Tea (serves four):

Ingredients:
- 12 Mint leaves(Pudina)
- 8 Basil Leaves(Tulsi)
- 4 Green cardamom (Elaichi)
- 2 gm Cinnamon (Dalchini)
- 20 gm Ginger (Adrak)
- 20 gm Jaggery (Gur)

Instructions:
- Take 4 cups of water in a tea pan
- Add all ingredients, simmer it for 10mins
- Add a dash of lemon juice and serve hot or cold

For those who are too lazy to collect the above ingredients (to make their own hunza tea) may order

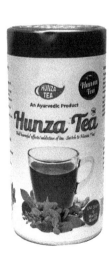

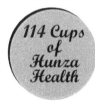

114 Cups of Hunza Health

₹ 400/-
(Including Courier charges)

You may place your order at:

Dynamic Memory Pvt. Ltd.
B-121, 2nd Floor, Green Fields,
Faridabad (Haryana)
Mobile No.:+91-9312286540,
E-mail: biswaroop@biswaroop.com

Log on to www.biswaroop.com/shop to buy products

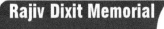
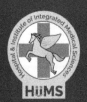
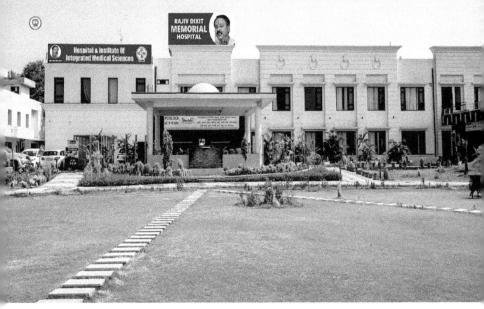

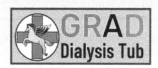
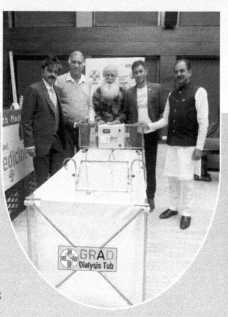
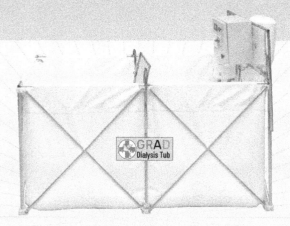
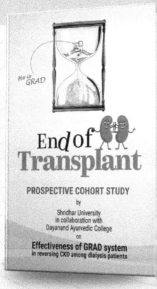

देश का सरदर्द करे दूर

2 SECONDS OIL

Headache
relief in 2 steps

Step 1 Open the cap **Step 2** Sniff the oil

न खाना   **न पीना**   **न लगाना**

सिर्फ सूंघकर करे सरदर्द को गायब

The box contains:

- 2 Seconds Oil bottle
- Certificate of Commitment
- Mini book 'देश का सिरदर्द करे दूर' 'Relieving Nation's Headache'

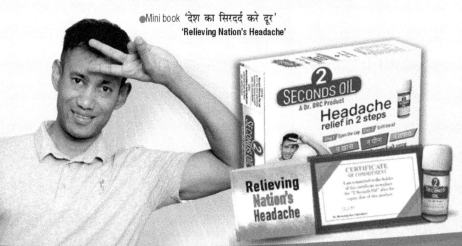

A Dr. BRC Product

To buy, go to
www.biswaroop.com/shop

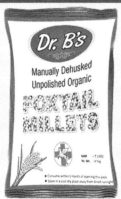

To visit Dr. BRC's
Banned Youtube Channel
go to
www.biswaroop.com/mydeletedyoutubechannel

&

for all new videos
go to

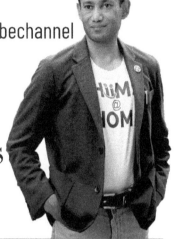

www.coronakaal.tv

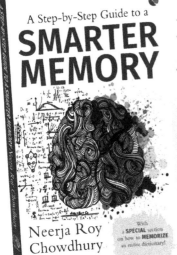
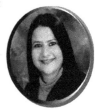

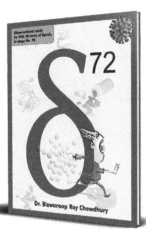
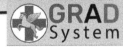

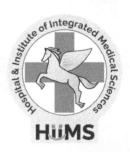
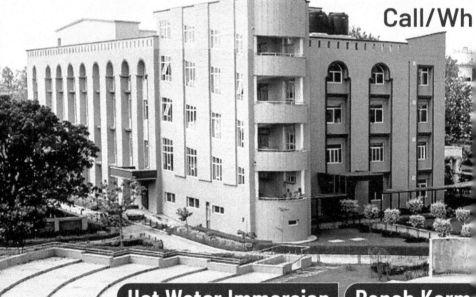

Camp with Dr. BRC

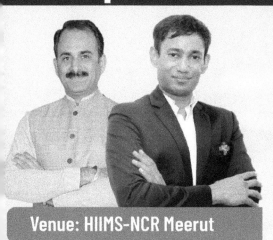

Diabetes
High B.P.
Heart Disease
Joint/Body Pains
Obesity
Swelling
Parkinson
Low Immunity
Constipation

Venue: HIIMS-NCR Meerut

ntegrated Medicine Hospital

pp: +91-7827710735

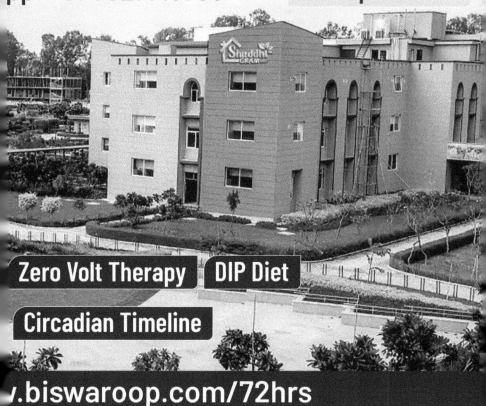

Zero Volt Therapy | **DIP Diet**

Circadian Timeline

.biswaroop.com/72hrs

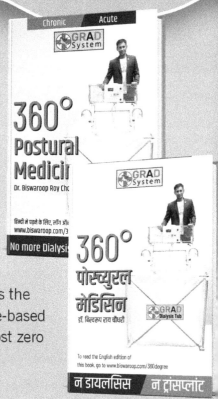

Ingram Content Group UK Ltd.
Milton Keynes UK
UKHW010718200423
420491UK00001B/74